SECTOR STRATEGY

Health, Nutrition, & Population

THE HUMAN DEVELOPMENT NETWORK
The World Bank Group
Washington, D.C.

Manufactured in the United States of America
First printing September 1997
4 5 6 04 03 02 01

The World Bank's Sector Strategy papers are designed to complement Country Assistance Strategies by providing a sectoral perspective on the Bank's comparative advantage, effectiveness, and priorities.

Each Sector Strategy paper provides a statement of the Bank's current strategy in a particular sector. These papers reflect the lessons learned about past Bank involvement in particular sectors based on internal and external evaluations. They also determine priorities for research, staffing, and policy work and contribute to the Country Assistance Strategy by identifying countries where particular sector issues loom large. They are intended to contribute to an ongoing dialogue among parties interested in promoting development in the sector.

The Sector Strategy papers will be produced by the Bank's Human Development Network, Poverty Reduction and Economic Management Network, Environment and Socially Sustainable Development Network, and Finance, Private Sector, and Infrastructure Network. It is hoped that the information provided in this and subsequent volumes of the series will prove valuable not only to Bank staff, but also to the international development community and to readers from client countries. These papers are viewed as a reflection of current thinking in the sector and a contribution to a dynamic dialogue among practitioners. It is hoped that they will promote constructive discussions leading to improvements in sector strategies over time.

The boundaries, colors, denominations, and other information shown on any map in this volume do not imply on the part of the World Bank Group any judgment on the legal status of any territory or the endorsement or acceptance of such boundaries.

Cover design by Supon Design Group, Washington, D.C.

Library of Congress Cataloging-in-Publication Data

Health, nutrition & population.
p. cm. — (Sector strategy)
ISBN 0-8213-4040-9
1. Nutrition policy. 2. Nutrition policy—Developing countries.
3. World health. I. World Bank. II. Title: Health, nutrition, and population. III. Series.
TX359.H43 1997
363.8—DC21 97-33552
CIP

Contents

Foreword

The World Bank's mandate is to work with governments to achieve sustainable progress in reducing poverty, promoting growth, and improving the quality of people's lives in developing countries. Current strategies to assist the poor rest on three mutually reinforcing pillars of development policy:

- expansion of opportunities through broad-based sustainable economic growth, especially to raise productivity and employment of the poor
- access by the poor to services that improve education, health, and nutrition outcomes, and that reduce fertility
- appropriate social safety net programs to protect especially vulnerable groups.

Good health, nutrition, and reproductive policies, and effective health services, are critical links in the chain of events that allow countries to break out of the vicious circle of poverty, high fertility, poor health, and low economic growth, replacing this with a virtuous circle of greater productivity, low fertility, better health, and rising incomes.

This Sector Strategy paper presents the World Bank's strategy in the health, nutrition, and population (HNP) area. The objectives of this paper are to:

- review major trends in the HNP sector, key development challenges, and the emerging consensus on reform strategies
- assess past and current Bank involvement in the HNP sector in low- and middle-income countries
- define a clear strategy to guide the Bank's future work in the HNP sector.

Many aspects of development policy that are not directly related to the health sector or to health services affect health, nutrition, and population outcomes. For example, education, water, sanitation, transport policy, and gun control affect health; agricultural and food policies affect nutrition; and multiple social and cultural dimensions affect population growth. Bank strategies toward the intersectoral determinants of health, nutrition, and population outcomes will be presented in forthcoming strategy papers.

In developing the Bank's strategy for the HNP sector, the following principles have been influential:

- a focus on the human dimension of development
- responsiveness to clients, especially the poor
- sound technical analysis and attention to outcomes
- recognition of the political dimensions of reforms
- respect for diversity in values and social choices
- the need for local ownership and partnerships.

The HNP Sector Strategy paper is the first major product of the HNP Family, which is part of the Bank's new Human Development Network, under the general guidance of the HNP Sector Board (see Annex D, Figure D.2). Its recommendations are closely linked to other Bank activities that are intended to improve operational effectiveness and contribute to each of five areas of responsibility of the HNP Sector Board: strategy, knowledge, staff development, quality assurance, and external partnerships.

An extensive consultative process has taken place to produce this document, involving interested staff in the Regions and the HNP Family as well as external partners. The strategy has been approved by senior management and endorsed by the Board.

The HNP Sector Strategy paper is not a final statement of the Bank's work in the HNP sector. This strategy will continue to evolve over time and will be revised.

David De Ferranti, HD Network Head & Director

Richard G.A. Feachem, HNP Director

Acknowledgments

This report was prepared by a team of technical specialists from the Health, Nutrition, and Population (HNP) Family of the Human Development (HD) Network of the World Bank under the guidance of the HNP Sector Board. The process involved staff and managers in other fields and sectors of the World Bank Group. The work was led by Alexander S. Preker, Principal Economist; Richard G.A. Feachem, HNP Director; and David De Ferranti, HD Network Head and Director. The document was edited by Madelyn Ross and document processing was done by Sancta E.M. Watley.

Summary

This HNP Sector Strategy paper is presented in three main sections, with supportive statistical annexes.

Development Challenges and Policy Directions

As described in Chapter I, this century has witnessed greater gains in health, nutrition, and population outcomes than at any other time in history.

These gains are partly the result of improvements in income and education, with accompanying improvements in nutrition, access to contraceptives, hygiene, housing, water supplies, and sanitation. They are also the result of new knowledge about the causes, prevention, and treatment of disease, and the introduction of policies that make interventions more accessible.

Despite past achievements, however, 2 million childhood deaths occur annually due to vaccine-preventable diseases; 200 million children under the age of five still suffer from malnutrition; 120 million couples still lack options in family planning; 7.5 million children die every year during the perinatal period; and 30 percent of the world is still without access to safe water and sanitation systems. In addition, disease patterns observed during the past century are rapidly changing.

As shown by broad international experience, the underlying threats to good health, nutrition, and population outcomes are well known, and affordable solutions are frequently available. But, because of weak government implementation capacity and market imperfections in the private sector, potentially effective policies and programs often fail.

Reform strategies to address these problems often require a redefinition of the role of the state, with greater government involvement in providing public health activities with large externalities, securing access to essential health services for the poor, providing information, supporting research and development (R&D) and medical education, regulating the sector, and securing adequate financing. They also require enhanced partnerships with non-governmental providers.

The Bank's Growing Engagement in the HNP Sector

Chapter II explains why investing in people is at the center of the Bank's development strategy, reflecting the fact that no country can secure sustainable economic growth or poverty reduction without healthy, well-nourished, and well-educated people. Since none of the international organizations can address today's complex health, nutrition, and population challenges alone, the Bank works closely with many other organizations. The Bank's comparative advantage is its global experience and ability to combine country-specific research and analysis with the mobilization of significant financial resources across many sectors.

Bank involvement in the HNP sector, which started in the early 1970s, initially helped countries strengthen and expand the infrastructure and supplies for basic programs. Although modest success was achieved through this approach, it became apparent that institutional and systemic changes were often needed for a sustained impact on outcomes for the poor, improved performance of health systems, and sustainable financing. The Country Assistance Strategy (CAS) is a key instrument for mobilizing the multi-sectoral involvement that is often needed to address systemic problems.

Since its first HNP loan in 1970, the Bank's activities in this sector have grown rapidly to the point where it is now the single largest external source of HNP financing in low- and middle-income countries. Today, there are 154 active and 94 completed Bank HNP projects, for a total cumulative value of US$13.5 billion in 1996 prices. This paper elaborates on the lessons learned from this experience and raises concerns about the recent decrease in analytical and policy work, a weakening in the presentation of HNP issues in the CAS, and the number of projects at risk.

The Bank's Strategy in the HNP Sector

Chapter III describes the Bank's enhanced commitment to the HNP sector during the period leading into the 21st century. The Bank's objectives in the HNP sector are to assist client countries to:

- ***improve the health, nutrition, and population outcomes of the poor***, and to protect the population from the impoverishing effects of illness, malnutrition, and high fertility
- ***enhance the performance of health care systems*** by promoting equitable access to preventive and curative health, nutrition, and population services that are affordable, effective, well managed, of good quality, and responsive to clients
- ***secure sustainable health care financing*** by mobilizing adequate levels of resources, establishing broad-based risk pooling mechanisms, and maintaining effective control over public and private expenditure.

The Bank's strategic direction in the HNP sector will continue to evolve in a dynamic way based on international best practice. The complexities of the HNP sector and changing approaches to health, nutrition, and population problems generally do not lend themselves to rigid policy prescriptions. Instead, policy advice and financial support will continue to be guided by country-specific approaches. This will be achieved through action in the following four areas:

Sharpening Strategic Directions. Governments will be encouraged to address each of the three HNP priorities outlined above, through decentralization, greater partnerships with non-governmental providers, and a more direct public involvement in securing sustainable financing. Governments will also be encouraged to address often neglected areas that have an impact on health, nutrition, and population outcomes such as rural and urban development, other broad-based population and social policies, education, control of tobacco and alcohol abuse, food and agricultural policies, environment, water supply, sanitation, and transportation.

The Bank's Country Assistance Strategy papers will be used as key instruments for delivering this message during high-level country dialogue. Greater efforts will be made to ensure that adequate budgets and staff time are allocated to the preparation of these important documents. Efforts will also be made to underpin lending with better research and analysis by reversing recent cutbacks in country-specific sector studies and linking the Bank's research agenda more closely to the HNP priorities. Staff will be encouraged to increase selectivity based on consistency with the HNP policy objectives, potential development impact, and political commitment by clients to significant reform.

Achieving Greater Impact. The quality of client services and client responsiveness will be enhanced by strengthening the HNP knowledge base; applying lessons learned more systematically; enhancing the quality of project preparation and the piloting of new approaches; improving supervision of existing projects; using a broader range of instruments; streamlining business processes and procurement procedures; and conducting client satisfaction surveys. Finally, a renewed effort will be made to strengthen monitoring and evaluation by developing better indicators and by integrating monitoring and evaluation into project designs.

Empowering Bank HNP Staff. Resolving three staffing issues will be a key priority for the new HNP Sector Board. Are there enough staff? Are their skills adequate to the tasks they must perform? Are they deployed effectively between headquarters and resident missions? This paper suggests how the Bank will be enhancing its capacity in these areas. An effort will be made to link training to the three strategic directions, include both Bank staff and clients in training events, increase participation by resident mission staff, and extend the target audience to sectors outside the HNP sector.

Building Partnerships. The Bank will continue to build relations with partners based on its comparative advantage and clear agreement on mutual roles, as it is now doing with WHO and UNAIDS. It will build on the past success in river blindness control and support other international health, nutrition, and population initiatives. Likely candidates include collaboration with African governments in a major effort to control the malaria epidemic, work with WHO and others to combat the pandemic of tuberculosis and to promote integrated management of childhood illness, and work with many partners to launch the Global Forum on Health Research.

Through such actions, the Bank expects to enhance its contribution to the global effort to improve human development during the first decade of the 21st century.

Acronyms and Initials

AfDB	African Development Bank
AIDS	Acquired Immune Deficiency Syndrome
AsDB	Asian Development Bank
CAS	Country Assistance Strategy
CODE	Committee on Development Effectiveness
DEC	Development Economics and Office of the Chief Economist
EAP	East Asia and Pacific Region of the World Bank
EBRD	European Bank for Reconstruction and Development
ECA	Europe and Central Asia Region of the World Bank
EDI	Economic Development Institute
ESW	Economic and Sector Work
EU	European Union
FAO	Food and Agriculture Organization of the United Nations
GDP	Gross Domestic Product
GNP	Gross National Product
HD	Human Development
HIV	Human Immunodeficiency Virus
HNP	Health, Nutrition, and Population
IBRD	International Bank for Reconstruction and Development
IDA	International Development Association
IDB	Inter-American Development Bank
IFC	International Finance Corporation
ILO	International Labour Organization
IMF	International Monetary Fund
LAC	Latin America and the Caribbean Region of the World Bank
LLC	Learning and Leadership Center
MIGA	Multilateral Investment Guarantee Agency
MNA	Middle East and North Africa Region of the World Bank
NGO	Non-Governmental Organization
OECD	Organization for Economic Cooperation and Development
OED	Operations Evaluation Department
PAHO	Pan American Health Organization
PPP	Purchasing Power Parity
PSD	Private Sector Development Department
QAG	Quality Assurance Group
R&D	Research and Development
SAS	South Asia Region of the World Bank
SECALs	Sector Adjustment Loans
SGP	Special Grants Program
SSA	Sub-Saharan Africa Region of the World Bank
TA	Technical Assistance
UNAIDS	Joint United Nations Programme on AIDS
UNDP	United Nations Development Programme
UNFPA	United Nations Population Fund
UNICEF	United Nations Children's Fund
WHO	World Health Organization

CHAPTER 1

Development Challenges and Policy Directions: A Changing World

Impressive Recent Gains in Outcomes

Advances in HNP during the past few decades are impressive. The increase in life expectancy and the decrease in fertility throughout the world have been greater in the past 40 years than during the previous 4,000 years. Furthermore, based on projections, the year 2000 will mark the mid-point of a century of global transition from high mortality and high fertility to low mortality and low fertility (see Figure 1.1 below and maps on Fertility Decline and Child Survival Goals in Annex G).

Unparalleled Improvements in Life Expectancy and Fertility Rates

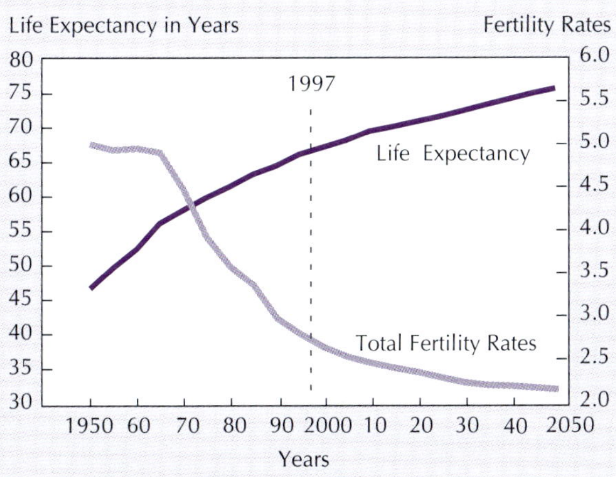

FIGURE 1.1

As described by the World Health Organization (WHO) in its *1996 World Health Report*, hundreds of millions of people in low- and middle-income countries are on the threshold of an era in which they will be safe from some of the world's most threatening diseases. According to the *1996 State of the World's Children*, by the United Nations Children's Fund (UNICEF), the proportion of children who now die before reaching age five is less than half the level in 1960. Immunization saves an estimated 3 million children annually. Better control of diarrhea saves over 1 million a year.

Economic progress during the past century has contributed significantly to health advances. Nutrition has improved not only from higher agricultural outputs per person and a greater ability to deal with local famines, but also from the introduction of a more varied diet. Child malnutrition rates in low- and middle-income countries are now 20 percent lower than they were 30 years ago, while certain nutrient deficiency diseases have almost disappeared in some countries.

Population growth rates are also slowing. The average number of children born to women of childbearing age (the total fertility rate) is now three, down from five in 1960. Some low- and middle-income countries have already reached replacement levels of around two children per family. Improvements in access to family planning, together with rising incomes and better education of girls and women, have facilitated this trend. Contraceptive use in low- and middle-income countries rose from 10 percent of married couples in the mid-1960s to 55 percent in 1990.

Origins of Good Health and Illness

Several factors influence the great variability in health, nutrition, and fertility still observed across population groups. These include:

- income levels and poverty;
- education, especially of girls and women;
- adequate food, clean water, and sanitation;
- culture and behavior; and
- health-related public policies and interventions.

Economic growth and reductions in poverty—with their impact on basic needs such as nutrition, better housing, and access to clean water and satisfactory sanitation—remain among the most powerful determinants of good health at low-income levels.

As shown in China, Costa Rica, and Sri Lanka, basic education of girls and women is also good for health. Educated individuals tend to adopt healthier lifestyles, make more efficient use of scarce resources such as food and health care, and avoid risks caused by the abuse of tobacco, alcohol, and illicit drugs. In most societies, norms regarding childbirth and child care, the status of women, personal hygiene, and sexual behavior exert powerful influences on health and are deeply rooted in local culture.

Population-based preventive services such as immunization play an important role in reducing the risk of illness, and curative services can greatly ameliorate the consequences of diseases and injuries when they occur. Other public policies can enhance health by promoting healthy environments and lifestyles, and regulating against dangerous or unhealthy activities by individuals and organizations. Successful public policies have helped reduce pollution in India, make road travel safer in Mexico, tighten gun control in the United Kingdom, improve water and sanitation systems in Turkey, and limit tobacco, alcohol, and illicit drug use in Indonesia. Stronger public policies are also still needed to eliminate female genital mutilation.

As a result of complex synergies among income levels, education, behavior, public policy, and health services, people all over the world live almost 25 years longer today than they would have at similar income levels in 1900 (see Figure 1.2).

Impressive Gains in Health at Similar Income Levels

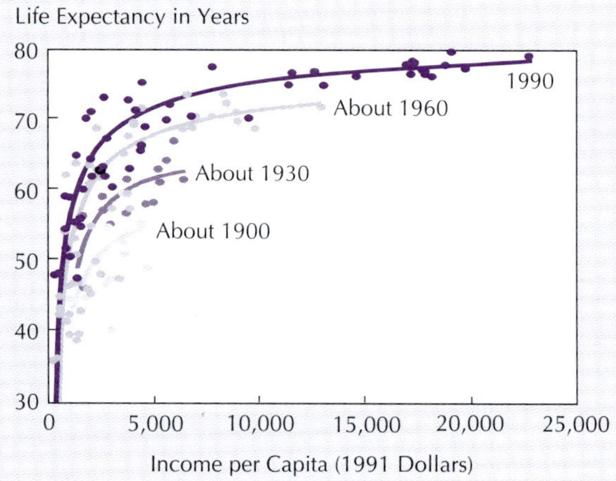

FIGURE 1.2

Impact on Quality of Life and Productivity

Good health contributes to the overall quality of life as well as to productivity. Many diseases are not fatal, but disabling. Some 200 million people throughout the world—90 percent in Sub-Saharan Africa—are infected with the parasitic schistosome worm, and 1 billion people suffer from anemia. The economic burdens of such illnesses include low productivity due to chronic fatigue and other symptoms, loss of income, out-of-pocket expenditure, and the cost of treatment.

Good health, by contributing to human capital, is essential to economic growth. For example, a single treatment of children in the West Indies for whipworm infection dramatically improved school learning. Labor productivity has increased with better iron and calorie intake in Indonesia and Kenya. Similarly, there is some evidence that reduced fertility rates and declining youth dependency ratios can have a positive impact on economic growth, if associated with domestic savings and investment in human capital.

Development Challenges

To preserve past gains and address future threats in an effective way, policymakers in low- and middle-income countries face difficult challenges caused by continued poverty, malnutrition, high fertility, and poor health; poor performance of many health systems; and inadequate and/or unsustainable health care financing.

Poverty, Malnutrition, High Fertility, and Poor Health

According to World Bank estimates, nearly one-quarter of the world's population—1.3 billion people—continue to live in absolute poverty, earning less than US$1 per day. The *1993 World Development Report: Investing in Health* estimated loss of healthy life from over 100 of the most common diseases and injuries. Of the total global disease burden, 93 percent is concentrated in low- and middle-income countries and nearly 60 percent is in China, India, and Sub-Saharan Africa.

The world's poorest populations live in the shadow of a group of old enemies—malnutrition, childhood infections, poor maternal/perinatal health, and high fertility (see Annex G map on Child Malnutrition). A total of 2 million deaths in children occur annually due to vaccine-preventable diseases; 200 million children under the age of five still suffer from malnutrition and anemia; 7.5 million children die every year during the perinatal period, primarily due to poor maternal health care; and 30 percent of the world is still without safe water and sanitation. Furthermore, because 120 million couples still lack options in family planning and receive poor maternal health services, one in every 48 women dies from pregnancy-related causes in low- and middle-income countries (585,000 deaths per year), compared with one in 4,000 in higher-income countries.

Intrauterine or early childhood exposure to undernutrition, micronutrient malnutrition (iron, iodine), or infection (diarrhea, malaria), often results in long term or irreversible retardation of physical and mental development. These conditions are particularly devastating to the poor, whose children enter adulthood and the workforce handicapped by early life experiences.

Rapid population growth is also a major development challenge in many poor countries and places a heavy burden on health care and social services. Even when fertility approaches replacement levels (close to two children per family), birth rates will continue to outstrip deaths for several decades because of the young population age structure that has resulted from past high fertility rates. The world's population could increase from 5.3 billion people in 1990 to over 10 billion in 2100. Most of this population growth will occur in poor countries.

The disease patterns of the past century are changing as population groups move from high mortality and fertility to low mortality and fertility. As a result, the share of global disease burden due to non-communicable diseases (mainly cardiovascular and neuro-psychiatric diseases, and cancers) is expected to increase from 36 percent in 1990 to 57 percent in 2020, while the burden due to infectious diseases, pregnancy, and perinatal causes is expected to drop from 49 to 22 percent. The emergence of new epidemics and drug resistant microbes and parasites will figure prominently among the remaining infectious diseases (see Annex G map on Malaria Distribution and Reported Drug Resistance).

Poor Performance of Many Health Systems

Much more research is needed to understand fully the factors that influence the performance of health systems. Partially as a result of differences in the effectiveness of broad social policies and health care systems, countries vary greatly in terms of the health, nutrition, and population outcomes they achieve at similar income levels (see Figure 1.3). As populations age and non-communicable diseases increase in low- and middle-income countries, there are obvious consequences for labor productivity, economic growth, and the cost of health care systems that must be adapted to new disease patterns and modes of intervention.

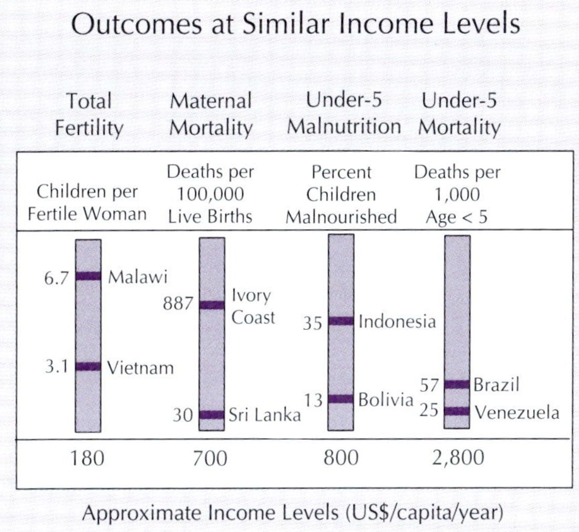

FIGURE 1.3

Differences in housing, access to clean water and satisfactory sanitation, education, income distribution, and culture all contribute to this variability, especially in low-income countries. But the use of knowledge about the determinants of poor health (e.g. the links between maternal nutrition and low birth weight, hygiene and infections, and smoking and heart disease) and implementation of effective preventive and curative health care (e.g. vaccinations, oral rehydration therapy, obstetrical care, and drug treatment of tuberculosis) are also important in explaining these differences.

Variability in Available Financing

Global spending on health care was about US$2,330 billion in 1994 (9 percent of global GDP), making it one of the largest sectors in the world economy. While low- and middle-income countries account for only 18 percent of world income and 11 percent of global health spending (US$250 billion or 4 percent of the GDP of developing countries), 84 percent of the world's population lives in these countries, and they shoulder 93 percent of the world's disease burden. The sheer size of the sector, and the fact that growth in health expenditure exceeds income growth, make it critical to understand the economic and health impact of health financing policies.

Health care behaves like a superior good in economic terms—poor countries spend much less than rich countries, both relative to GDP and on a per capita basis (see Figure 1.4). In addition, a country's public expenditure on health care rises with income both in absolute and relative terms. This is reflected in the large differences in the proportion of national GDP spent on health—from under 1 percent in some countries to 15 percent in the United States. Per capita health expenditures (public and private) vary almost 1,000-fold among countries—from around US$3 to $5 per capita per year in some low-income countries such as Mali to $3,600 in the United States (the ratio would be 225 using PPP-adjusted dollars).

The Sub-Saharan Africa (SSA), South Asia (SAS), and East Asia and Pacific (EAP) regions spend the least on health care in absolute terms (see map on Health Expenditures in Annex G), and some countries are spending less over time. Low tax collection capacity and low personal income contribute to these trends. Lack of financing usually translates into low levels of capital stock such as beds, and of human resources such as doctors and nurses. Even where capital stock is more adequate on a national basis, inequitable resource distribution may result in poor access to services by the poor, such as in the Middle East and North Africa (MNA) region.

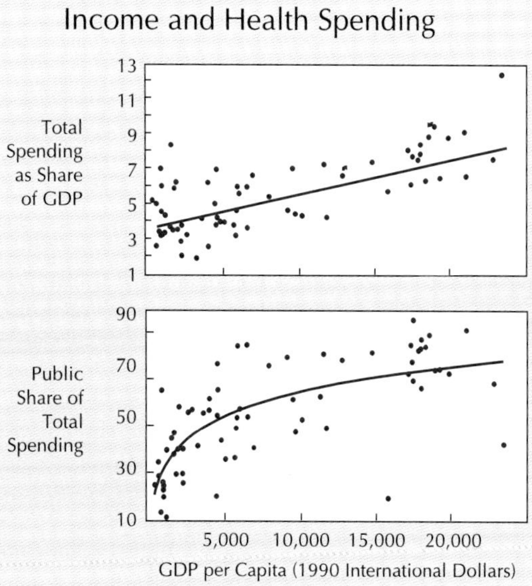

FIGURE 1.4

Recently a growing number of countries face a different challenge—rapidly rising health expenditures in both the public and private sector. Some countries have increased health spending from 3-5 percent of GDP to 8-10 percent of GDP in only a few years. Argentina now spends a higher share of GDP on health than Canada, which for years ranked second only to the United States. Often public funding is forced above what is fiscally sustainable, and too often additional spending goes to ineffective, inefficiently managed, and low quality care. Increased spending on health care alone does not necessarily increase health, nutrition, and population outcomes. Attention to population-based approaches and broad public health approaches are often needed before outcomes are influenced.

The reasons for these increases in health care expenditure include rapid escalation in the cost of new medical technology, the epidemiological transition in disease patterns (increase in chronic diseases and re-emerging or new communicable diseases), rising popular expectations, and the growth of fee-for-service medicine and third party insurance.

At a global annual growth rate for GDP of 3.5 percent, health care expenditure will increase by about US$82 billion a year worldwide, or US$9 billion a year in low- and middle-income countries at current rates of growth. In principle, this is enough money to pay for essential population-based preventive and curative services for the 900 million of the world's estimated 1.3 billion poor who still do not have adequate access to these services. However, if current trends persist, many of these resources will go to those who already have access and use services, rather than to the poor.

Major Policy Directions

The underlying threats to good health, nutrition, and population outcomes are well known, and affordable solutions are frequently available. But because of weak government implementation capacity and market imperfections in the private sector (especially with respect to public goods and activities with large externalities), recommended policies often fail to benefit the poor, fail to improve the impact of health systems, and fail to secure sustainable financing for the sector. This section provides a framework for understanding recent changes in the role of the state, and reforms that many countries are adopting in the HNP sector.

The Changing Roles of the State and Private Sectors

Throughout most of history, people used home remedies, private doctors and other health care workers, and nongovernmental hospitals when they were ill. Often only the rich could afford such care and the range of effective treatment was limited. Today, in low-income countries—where public revenues are scarce (often less than 20 percent of GDP) and institutional capacity in the public sector is weak—the financing and delivery of HNP services is largely in the private sector. In many of these countries, large segments of the poor still have no access to basic or effective care for a variety of reasons discussed below.

In most developed countries—and many middle-income countries—governments have become central to social policy and health care. This involvement by the public sector is justified on both theoretical and practical grounds to improve: (a) **equity,** by securing access by the population to health, nutrition, and reproductive services; and (b) **efficiency,** by correcting for market failures, especially when there are significant externalities (public goods) or serious information asymmetries (health insurance).

One of the clearest cases for strong government intervention in the HNP sector can be made when there are large externalities (the benefits to society are greater than the sum of benefits to individuals). This is true in the case of clean water, sanitation services, vector control, food safety measures, and a range of public health interventions (e.g. immunization, family planning, maternal and perinatal health care, control of infectious diseases, and control of tobacco, alcohol, and illicit drug abuse). Medical education and R&D are two other areas for active government intervention.

Private voluntary health insurance is one area which is particularly prone to a number of market imperfections, many of which relate to information asymmetries. While insurance may succeed in protecting some people against selected risks, it usually fails to cover everyone willing to subscribe to insurance plans and it often excludes those who need health insurance the most or who are at greatest risk of illness. This happens because insurers have a strong incentive to enroll only healthy or low-cost clients (risk selection or cream-skimming). Private insurers also have incentives to exclude costly conditions or to minimize their financial risk through the use of benefit caps and exclusions. This limits protection against most expensive and catastrophic illnesses.

Because of these factors, individuals who know they are at risk of illness have a strong incentive to conceal their underlying medical condition (adverse selection). Individuals who are—or at least think they are—healthy will often try to pay as low premiums as possible. This prevents insurers from raising the funds needed to cover the expenses incurred by sicker or riskier members. Worse, the healthy may even deliberately under-insure themselves, in the hope that free or highly subsidized care will be available when they become ill (free-riding). When third-party insurers pay, both patients and providers have less incentive to be concerned about costs, and some may even become careless about maintaining good health. This leads not only to more care being used (the reason for insurance), but also to less effective care, or care that would not be needed if people maintained good health (moral hazard).

In addition to insurance market failure, private consumers are also at the mercy of medical providers who charge what the market will bear. Without good regulations and quality control systems, patients can spend a significant amount of their personal income on ineffective care. The poor and less well educated are particularly vulnerable to unscrupulous profit seeking by private providers, due to information asymmetries.

The main actions taken by governments to correct for such market failures, from least to greatest intervention, include: providing information to encourage behavior changes needed for long-term improvements in health, nutrition, and population outcomes; enforcing regulations and incentives to influence public and private sector activities; issuing mandates to indirectly finance or provide services; financing or providing subsidies to pay for services or influence prices; and direct public production of preventive and curative health services.

Both economic principles and empirical evidence suggest that a mixture of public and private involvement leads to the best results in the HNP sector. Neither sector is effective by itself—each needs the other. Both too much and too little involvement by either sector are often associated with problems.

Unfortunately, in low- and middle-income countries, weak institutional capacity to deal effectively with regulatory problems in the private sector often causes governments to become excessively involved in the direct production of health services. Such over-involvement in public production is typically associated with insufficient government involvement in: providing information about personal hygiene, healthy life-styles, and appropriate use of health care; regulating the private sector; financing essential health services, especially for the poor; and securing access to public goods with large externalities for the whole population. The reforms that are needed to strike an optimal balance at various income levels differ in the case of delivery systems and financing. This will be discussed in more detail below.

Recent Reform Strategies

Recent dissatisfaction with poor health, nutrition, and population outcomes, the low quality of health care in both public and private facilities, and the lack of sustainable financing and/or cost escalation have led to a wave of health care reforms throughout the world. (See the *At A Glance* tables in Annex A for clusters of countries that perform poorly in each of these three priority areas.)

Improving HNP Outcomes for the Poor

The majority of the world's 1.3 billion people identified by the Bank as living in absolute poverty, with incomes of less than US$1 per day, live in countries where a sizable proportion of the population still lacks adequate access to safe drinking water and sanitation, adequate nutrition, basic shelter, basic education, family planning, and essential health services.

In poor countries, the design of policies and programs to ensure access to essential HNP services—whether implemented through public or private channels—is an absolute priority (See Annex B for a discussion of the *UN Basic Social Services for All* initiative and Annex C for a more detailed description of selected essential HNP interventions). Often non-targeted and targeted strategies must be undertaken in parallel.

Non-Targeted Approaches. The experience in developed and middle-income countries is that universal access is one of the most effective ways to provide health care for the poor. But non-targeted approaches can also be wasteful. Some low-income countries spend as much as 4 percent of GDP on publicly-funded food subsidies with little impact on the nutrition of the poor. In low-income countries, non-targeted approaches often have to be restricted to a very limited range of public health and food fortification programs, and a few essential health services, to be financially viable.

Targeted Approaches. It is possible to ensure that essential programs reach those who need them most through use of careful targeting. The following four approaches are particularly relevant to the HNP sector in low- and middle-income countries:

- *Focus specifically on the poor individuals or households most vulnerable to illness, malnutrition, and high fertility*, by applying a means test to identify the neediest and providing free or subsidized services to only those qualifying for preferential access on this basis. In most low-income countries this technique is not administratively feasible on a large scale.
- *Focus on poor regions within a country or on population groups that are particularly vulnerable to poverty* (e.g., women, children, and ethnic minorities). At the global level, most of the world's 1.3 billion poor live in South Asia, Sub-Saharan Africa, and a few countries in other regions (see Annex A for country groupings). Within countries, the emphasis can be on the states, rural areas, and urban areas where the poor live, or on specific sub-groups within these areas—such as when nutrition programs are targeted at mothers and young children in disadvantaged areas.
- *Emphasize health, nutrition, and reproductive problems of the poor.* The old enemies of the poor—malnutrition, communicable diseases, childhood illnesses, high fertility, and maternal and perinatal conditions—can be specifically targeted in this way (see Figure 1.5). More than half of the disease burden in Sub-Saharan Africa and South Asia can be addressed effectively through local adaptation of interventions such as immunization, food fortification, targeted nutrition programs, integrated management of childhood illness, family planning, maternal and perinatal health, and school health (see Annex C). As populations age, non-communicable conditions and injuries increase rapidly. The poor and less well educated are particularly vulnerable to the adverse effects of mass marketing of tobacco, alcohol products, and unhealthy foods.

- *Give greatest attention to the types of service providers from whom the poor receive most of their care.* This often requires upgrading and extending the health, nutrition, and reproductive services (public and private) in low density rural areas and urban slums. This would include improving the supply of consumables and drugs, the management of facilities, and the skills of staff.

Communicable Diseases: A Major Killer Among the Poor

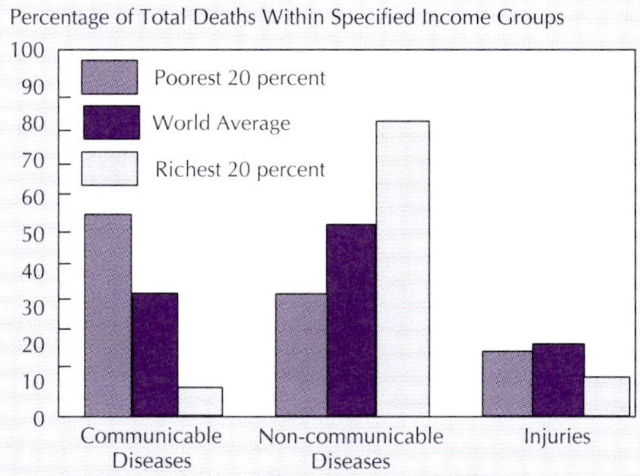

FIGURE 1.5

Enhancing Performance of HNP Services

Designing effective policies and reforms to improve the performance of both government-run and private health systems has bedeviled both rich and poor countries over the past decade.

Reforms in Public Delivery Systems. Much remains to be learned about how to make publicly-owned health systems more effective. The following public sector reforms are often needed:

- *Improving equity in access* to a range of preventive and clinical services through: (i) reduced geographic, financial, cultural, and other barriers; (ii) interventions that address conditions that are frequent and inexpensive to treat (at least for the poor); (iii) interventions that are less frequent, more damaging to health, and costlier but still within a country's means.
- *Raising efficiency in the use of scarce resources* through improvements in policymaking, governance, encouraging market incentives, management, decentralization, and accountability.
- *Improving the effectiveness of interventions* through improved clinical and management skills, design of basic preventive and clinical packages, treatment protocols, technology review panels, limited drug formularies, training, and research on the efficacy and cost of different interventions.
- *Raising the quality of care* through incentives, improved information, training, accreditation systems (for HNP staff and establishments), peer reviews, inspection systems, and routine surveillance.
- *Maximizing consumer satisfaction* through increased choice and attention to client surveys.

The Limits to Public Sector Reforms. Public sector reforms of government-run health services are often not enough to correct the deep-rooted problems that plague these systems. Despite years of effort and investment, many government-run systems continue to be underfinanced and perform poorly. In many cases they do not provide the desired access, effectiveness, efficiency, and quality. Even in the poorest of countries, patients frequently turn to private providers. Those who can afford to pay the price can sometimes find the quality of care that they seek. The poor often fall prey to cheap and ineffective remedies provided by unscrupulous profit seekers in an unregulated market place.

More Balanced Public/Private Mix. Although the optimal balance between public and private involvement varies considerably from one country to another, and is different in the case of financing from that in the case of service delivery, many recent reforms focus on correcting inequities and inefficiencies that occur when the balance between government and private sector roles becomes excessively distorted in one direction or another (see Annex A for a ranking of low- and middle-income countries that are at either extreme of the public/private mix and the left box in Figure 1.6 for distorted government roles).

Governments in countries that have introduced successful reforms often increase their role in providing information, regulations, mandates, and financing. While fostering a more balanced participation by NGOs, local communities, and the private sector in the service delivery systems, governments in these countries have shifted their attention and scarce resources to: securing access by the whole population to services with large externalities (preventive public health services); providing basic health, nutrition, and population services for the poor; and assuming sectoral oversight responsi-

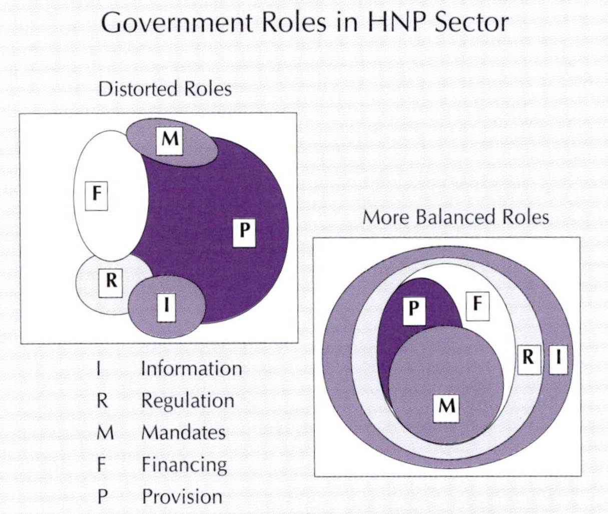

FIGURE 1.6

bility for financing, medical education, R&D, and quality control (see right box in Figure 1.6 and discussion on financing in the section below).

The *initial wave* in reforms of the state often includes a divestiture of state assets, or privatization, which is concentrated on commercial enterprises. Success in this area leads to a *second wave*—the divestiture of public infrastructure and utilities. Finally, as confidence is gained in these two areas, divestiture of state assets continues, with a focus on non-governmental and private management and investment in health, education, and pensions systems—the *third wave*.

As seen in other sectors that have gone through this process and the health sector in the OECD, greater non-governmental participation does not necessarily imply the sale of public assets. Instead, it can involve initiatives that allow greater private sector participation, such as private co-financing, management contracts, outsourcing, and trusts. Divestiture of social assets requires an enhanced, rather than a diminished, regulatory role by governments in quality assurance, securing fair competition, and preventing abuses.

Improving Health Care Financing

In health care financing, blind faith in the market is no more likely to resolve the complex problems that face the health sector than a naive belief in government. The approaches used to pool risks, secure sustainable financing, contain costs, and balance the budget in the HNP sector are different from approaches used to enhance partnerships with non-governmental and private providers of services (see Annex A for groupings of countries that have problems securing adequate levels of financing or containing costs).

Pooling of risks. Some people are much sicker than others. Sharing of risks across population groups is a fundamental aspect of social protection in the HNP sector. Furthermore, people use health care most during childhood, the childbearing years, and old age—when they are the least productive economically. Income smoothing across the life-cycle can, therefore, also contribute to social protection in the HNP sector.

Yet as in 19th century Europe, when health care was still in a primitive stage of development, direct out-of-pocket health expenditure continues to be a distinctive feature of many low- and middle-income countries. Household payments can account for as much as 80 percent of total health expenditures because of: nontrivial user fees charged in public facilities (official and unofficial); high copayments required in health insurance schemes; and use of private health services (hospitals, clinics, diagnostics, medicines, and health care providers). This undermines the social protection that could be provided by the HNP sector even in low-income settings.

Experience has shown that strong action is needed by the public sector to take advantage of the substantial resources that can be mobilized through private channels, while at the same time ensuring social protection for vulnerable groups. Because of cost and the pronounced market failure that occurs in private health insurance, this is not a viable option for risk pooling at the national level in low- and middle-income countries.

Securing Adequate Levels of Financing. Strong, direct government intervention is needed in most countries to finance public health activities and essential health, nutrition, and reproductive services, as well as to provide protection against the impoverishing effects of catastrophic illness.

In low-income countries, total government revenues may constitute 20 percent or less of GDP. A country with a per capita income in the range of US$300 to US$800 would have to spend in the range of 1.5 to 3 percent of GDP (equivalent to 7.5 to 15 percent of government revenues) to finance a minimum level of preventive and essential clinical services. Many low-income countries spend less than this. Governments in these countries may need to mobilize additional financing from community sources and international donors to pay for

Low-Income Countries Have Weak Capacity to Raise Revenues

- Governments in many countries often raise less than 20% of GDP in public revenues; and
- The tax structure in many low-income countries is often regressive.

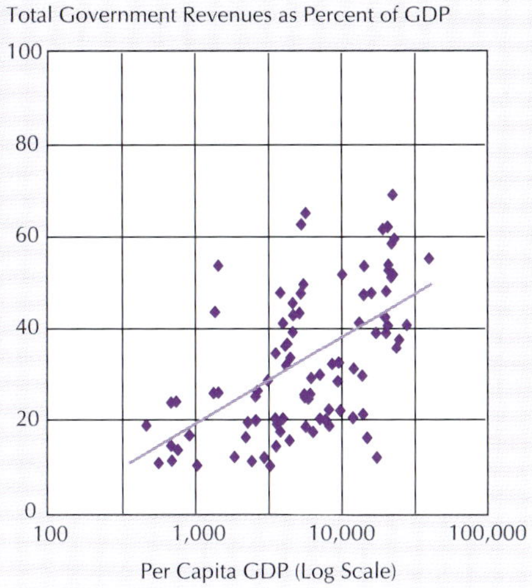

FIGURE 1.7

public health interventions with large externalities and essential programs for the poor (see Figure 1.7).

In middle-income countries, with per capita incomes above US$800, even at low tax collection rates, governments may choose to spend as much as 3 to 5 percent of GDP on health care. This is usually more than sufficient to pay for care that goes well beyond essential preventive and clinical services for the poor.

In these countries, other considerations become important, such as tailoring the mix of broad-based financing instruments to each country's individual circumstances. Critical factors in this respect would include equity and efficiency in collection mechanisms, administrative simplicity, budget mechanisms, cost containment, willingness to pay, affordability of the benefit package, and stability in the underlying macro-economic environment. It also involves ensuring that a large share of financing derives from a prepaid source of revenues (risk pooling through general revenues, and/or social or mandated health insurance that is community rated) to avoid the equity and efficiency problems associated with extensive reliance on user charges.

Containing Costs and Fiscal Discipline. Even in low- and middle-income countries, a significant share of national product and public resources is spent on health care. Although there are no fixed upper limits, fiscal concern may be warranted if total health spending is greater than 6 to 7 percent of GDP or if it is rising rapidly, since public funds are often involved. In too many countries, high expenditure levels involve public money spent on ineffective services that benefit only a few, while large segments of the population still do not have adequate access to essential care. In cases where expenditure control becomes an issue, governments have recourse to three broad types of policies:

- Policies that contain costs in the public sector through supply, demand, and price control strategies;
- Policies that regulate the private sector, discourage the use of indemnity insurance, and encourage capitation payments rather than fee-for-service; and
- Policies that strengthen monitoring and tracking of health expenditure patterns (using health accounts).

Improving Budget Practices and Resource Allocation. Unfortunately, in a large number of low- and middle-income countries, one of the key issues relating to health care financing is neither lack of adequate resources nor run-away expenditures. Rather, problems in health care financing often result from poor budget practices in the sector, including a habit of deficit financing and a misallocation of scarce resources on ineffective care. Three policies help countries balance their budget:

- Ensuring that income from all sources exceeds expected aggregate recurrent expenditure levels by a margin (often 3 to 5 percent) that is sufficient to cover depreciation, and major maintenance;
- Enforcing clear sanctions against budget overruns and the accumulation of irreducible debt; and
- Allocating a large part of the budget envelope to effective interventions that improve outcomes.

The Bank's role in helping countries address these issues and reforms is discussed in Chapter II.

CHAPTER II

The Bank's Role: Growing Engagement and Learning

Rationale For Bank Involvement

Investing in people is at the center of the World Bank's development strategy as it moves into the 21st century, reflecting the fact that no country can secure sustainable economic growth or poverty reduction without a healthy, well nourished, and educated population.

What Developing Countries Say They Need

To address the HNP poverty agenda, improve the performance of health services, and secure affordable and sustainable financing for the sector, most countries say they need assistance from the international community in the form of both broad international experience, and country-focused policy advice and financing.

Yet responding directly to client demand in the HNP sector is not straightforward. First, it is necessary to reconcile the divergent views of the various interest groups—the Bank's clients (typically the ministries of health and finance), stakeholders (local communities, health care providers, and insurance companies), beneficiaries (patients, the poor, women, children, and other vulnerable groups), and other development partners.

Second, many countries have health, nutrition, and population problems precisely because governments introduced the wrong policies in the past. Often they failed to implement good policies and were unable to harness non-governmental resources effectively. Even small changes in outcome may take as long as 10 to 15 years to realize, extending beyond the average government's term and commitment to reform.

Finally, when financial assistance to the HNP sector is sought in the form of credits and loans, this strategy must be carefully balanced with the medium-term returns to such investments and the opportunity cost of not investing in other spheres of the economy that impact on health, nutrition, and population outcomes.

Role of the International Community

None of the international organizations can address today's complex health, nutrition, and reproductive challenges alone. This is especially true since overseas development assistance from the world's richest countries has now dropped to less than 0.3 percent of their combined GDP—its lowest level in 20 years.

The Bank works with many other international organizations (FAO, ILO, UNAIDS, UNDP, UNFPA, UNICEF, WHO), regional banks (AsDB, AfrDB, EBRD, and IDB), the EU, bilateral organizations and NGOs, and the private sector. The Bank's collaboration and partnership with many of these agencies has improved, but there is still room for further strengthening.

The Bank's strengths are its global expertise, its multisectoral macro-level country focus, and the ability to mobilize large financial resources (either directly or through partnerships). For technical expertise in specific areas of the HNP sector such as disease control, the Bank seeks assistance from its UN sister agencies and other international partners.

The Bank's Involvement in HNP

The Bank's role in the HNP sector during the past 25 years has been one of growing engagement and learning in two key areas.

- First, the Bank has contributed to the generation and dissemination of global knowledge on health, nutrition, and population issues through regional and global studies, operational research and analysis, and shared international experiences.
- Second, underpinned by the knowledge base that it has accumulated in this work, the Bank has been instrumental in catalyzing development change at the country level through its main nonlending activities (described below) and its financing instruments.

Generation and Dissemination of Global Knowledge

Cross-Cutting Policy Studies

Many of the Bank's past policy studies in the HNP sector have focused on the role of the state and non-governmental sectors in addressing the health, nutrition, and population needs of the poor, performance of health systems, and sustainable financing.

Noteworthy early Bank policy papers include: (a) the *1970 Sectoral Programs and Policies Paper*, which included recommendations on population policies; (b) the *1973 Sector Program Paper* on Bank nutrition activities; and (c) the *1975 Health Sector Policy Paper.*

The *1980 Health Sector Policy Paper* was the first attempt to set out a solid rationale for free-standing Bank investments in the health sector, drawing links between health sector activities, poverty alleviation, and family planning. The influential *1980 World Development Report on Human Resources* highlighted the importance of the health sector, along with education and social protection, to poverty alleviation strategies.

The *1984 World Development Report: Population and Development* emphasized the role of governments in reducing mortality and fertility. The 1987 policy study, *Financing Health Services in Developing Countries: An Agenda for Reform*, tackled the policy themes of inefficient and inequitable public spending on health care and recurrent cost financing.

The theme of the role of governments was repeated in the Bank's seminal piece on the HNP sector, the 1993 *World Development Report: Investing in Health*. This report has already had a substantial impact on national and international debates on health policies in low- to middle-income countries, and on priorities for the Bank's work. The 1992 report on *Development and the Environment*, the 1996 report on *From Plan to Market*, and the 1997 report on *The Role of the State* also dealt with HNP issues.

In addition to such major policy reports, the Bank has also published many books, technical notes, and working papers that deal with HNP issues—163 such studies were published by the end of FY96. Efforts have been made recently to experiment with shorter, more focused, and less resource-intensive products as well as out-sourcing some of the research (e.g., the IFC's 1997 *Private Hospital Investment Study*).

Operational Research and Analysis

About US$20 million out of the approximately US$80 million allocated to the Bank's Special Grants Program (SGP) in FY96 went to HNP sector activities. Recent HNP-related programs supported by the SGP include the Special Program of Research, Development, and Training in Human Reproduction, the WHO/UNDP/World Bank Tropical Diseases Research Program, the International Health Policy Program, the WHO Ad Hoc Review on Health Research, and the Global Micronutrient Initiative.

Country-specific research and analysis of HNP issues supported through Bank loans and credits has recently ranged between approximately US$50 and US$75 million per year. This is 5 to 6 percent of total lending and by far the largest source of external research funding for HNP in client countries.

The Bank's Policy Research Department has several staff working on HNP-related issues and has conducted a number of HNP studies in recent years. Its HNP research expenditure is about US$1.1 million per year or 8 percent of that department's total research budget of US$14.5 million. A major recent project has been the preparation of a policy research report on *AIDS and Development*. The Research Advisory Department also supports competitive research projects in HNP.

Shared International Experiences

The Bank's Economic Development Institute (EDI) provides training and seminars for senior policymakers in client countries on HNP issues. The Learning and Leadership Center (LLC) of the Bank focuses on training for Bank staff. The HNP Family of the HD Network, established in 1996, is leading HNP knowledge management work in the Bank. All three groups are making increasing use of partnerships and electronic technologies to maximize their impact.

The EDI-HD Network flagship course on *Health Sector Reform and Sustainable Financing* in the fall of 1997—which involves six regionally-based partner institutes—will focus on the economic, political economy, and institutional issues central to HNP reforms. During the past two years, the LLC-HD Network training week has provided staff with intensive training focused on topical issues in the HNP sector.

International conferences and scientific meetings organized by both the Bank and other organizations also provide training opportunities for Bank staff and client countries. The Bank was a participant in the 1990 UNICEF-led World Summit on Children in New York, the 1991 International Meeting of Partners for Safe Motherhood in Washington, DC, the 1994 International Conference on Population and Development in Cairo, the 1995 World Conference on Women in Beijing, and the 1996 International Conference on Early Childhood Development in Atlanta. In addition, the Bank organized and hosted the 1997 International Conference on Innovations in Health Financing in Washington, DC.

The Bank encourages its client countries to participate in such international conferences and scientific meetings in an effort to strengthen institutional capacity and to provide an opportunity for shared learning.

Areas for Improvement as a Global Knowledge Broker

Although many Bank policy studies have had an impact on development, concern has been expressed recently that some lack operational relevance, that most take a long time to develop, and that they are resource-intensive both in terms of direct cost and the opportunity cost of staff drawn away from other work. Research and training—undertaken directly by the Bank or supported indirectly through loans and grants—must also remain relevant to the emerging development priorities in the HNP sector, and to the operational needs of staff and client countries. The research undertaken through lending is typically not designed or supervised by staff with training or skills in research. And recent budget stringency and operational pressures often make it difficult for staff to take full advantage of the training opportunities available at the Bank and elsewhere.

Catalyzing Change at the Country Level

It is at the country level that the Bank's global experience, multi-sectoral macro-level country focus, and financial resources are brought together in an effort to catalyze development change in the HNP sector as in other sectors. Both the Bank's non-lending activities, in the form of country-specific economic and sector work (ESW), and its financing in the form of loans, credits, and grants, are used to promote needed systemic reforms and maximize the impact of policy advice.

Country-Specific Policy Advice and Client Dialogue

The Country Assistance Strategy (CAS) has become the Bank's central vehicle for development assistance in low- and middle-income countries. It provides an opportunity to highlight stubborn cross-sectoral issues, and to establish critical links between the HNP sector and a country's poverty and fiscal agendas. Since the CAS sets the agenda for the Bank's future work (both studies and lending) in the HNP sector, inputs based on country-specific sectoral analysis and assessments of the effectiveness of past lending operations are a critical part of the CAS process.

The FY96 Malawi CAS provides a good example of how key issues relating to poor health and the lack of a healthy environment (lack of sanitation, potable water, basic education, and adequate income) can be presented in the CAS. Reproductive health and human resource development were identified as priority areas for the country's future growth and development. Based on this analysis, the CAS presented a strategy for reform in the HNP sector, which was linked to the macro-framework and shortcomings in the government's current health, nutrition, and population policies.

In the future, HNP staff will work more closely with other staff from the HD Network and country teams to ensure adequate links between the HNP sector and the Bank's poverty alleviation and macro-economic strategies. Currently, the analytical framework used to underpin most CAS recommendations does not include quantitative variables for human capital or labor productivity, both of which are influenced by HNP outcomes and educational attainment. Furthermore, reluctance to address politically sensitive topics is often a key reason for not addressing deep-rooted systemic issues that impact on the HNP sector. These problems undermine the Bank's comparative advantage as a multi-sectoral agency and diminish the impact of its macro-level focus on the HNP sector.

For example, many CASs do not address financial sustainability and manpower issues in the HNP sector as an integral part of public finance and civil service reforms. Furthermore, the CAS could be more explicit about discouraging client countries from subsidizing unhealthy agricultural products and wasting public resources on untargeted food compensation programs. Finally, given the emerging chronic disease epidemic, client countries should be encouraged to use taxation instruments to combat tobacco abuse.

Most of the Bank's policy advice in the HNP sector relies on shared international best practice and adapting applicable lessons to country-specific settings. For example, the approach to population issues is largely guided by the recommendations of the 1994 International Conference on Population and Development in Cairo (see Annex B). A similar approach is used in the disease control and nutrition areas. This is considered the best way to address the complex issues faced in the HNP sector. In the case of tobacco, international best practice is reflected in the 1992 Bank policy of not supporting any tobacco production, processing, or marketing, while actively encouraging tobacco control (Operational Directive 4.76).

Issues relating to the political economy of reform, behavior changes, and social marketing require more attention in the future. A prerequisite for improvement in this area is to make staff more sensitive to the practical constraints faced by politicians and bureaucrats in countries trying to implement HNP reforms.

Country-Specific Analytical Studies in HNP Sector

Country-specific analytical studies—also known as economic and sector work (ESW)—are an important part of the Bank's non-lending work in HNP. These studies allow Bank staff to learn about the health, nutrition, and population issues and investment needs in individual client countries. They are a critical input for both the CAS and client dialogue. Many client countries with only moderate financial needs seek to gain access to the technical expertise mobilized during the Bank's investment project cycle.

In addition to the 210 country-specific sector studies and Staff Appraisal Reports completed by the end of FY96, hundreds of shorter working documents and country strategy papers have been written on selected HNP topics. Such studies have recently been done on Argentina, Brazil, Chile, China, Jordan, Kyrgyz Republic, India, Malawi, Mexico, and Tunisia.

One assessment of the impact of the Bank's activities shows that most of the foreign aid to the HNP sector simply substitutes for government spending. The real source of aid effectiveness in HNP is, therefore, the reforms resulting from policy advice that accompany lending, not the loans themselves. In light of this finding, past and future cuts in the budget and staff-time allocated to analytical work are a worrisome trend (see Figure 2.1).

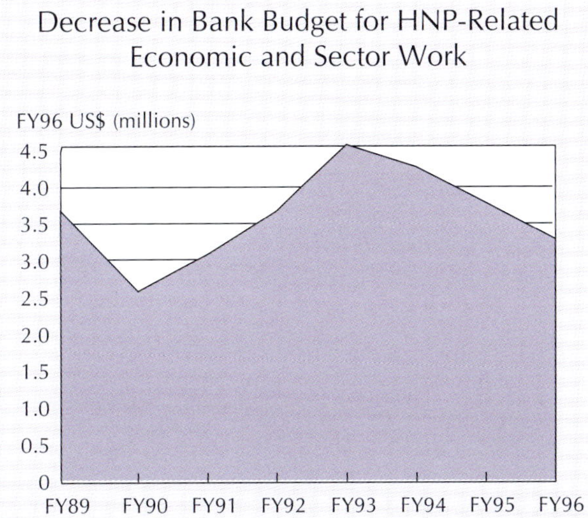

FIGURE 2.1

The Bank's past analytical work in HNP did not pay sufficient attention to the political economy of reform and its economic, regulatory, and institutional underpinnings. More work is also needed to translate international experience with reform into practical solutions at the country and local level. In the past, even when best practice information was available in some of these areas within the Bank's vast knowledge base, this information was not always readily accessible to Bank staff.

Financing (Loans, Credits, and Grants)

Bank financial support for the Human Development (HD) sector began with education lending in the 1960s. This was followed by lending to the HNP sector in the 1970s and 1980s, and later broadened to include social investment funds, employment funds, training programs, social transfers (pensions and safety nets), and early childhood development.

By the end of FY96, 24 percent of the annual US$21 billion in new Bank loans was directed to the HNP, education, and social protection sectors. In addition to these direct human development activities, an additional 23 percent of total Bank lending is devoted to the agriculture, water supply and sanitation, environment, and rural/urban development sectors, which also impact on health, nutrition, and population outcomes.

Since the Bank's first loan of US$2 million to family planning activities in Jamaica in 1970, its activities in the HNP sector have grown to the point where it is now the largest single external financier in low- to middle-income countries, with a cumulative portfolio value of over US$13.5 billion in 1996 prices (see Figure 2.2). In 1976 the first nutrition loan went to Brazil, and in 1981 Tunisia was the first country to borrow for a project to expand basic health services.

Cumulative Growth in HNP Lending and Projects (1996 prices)

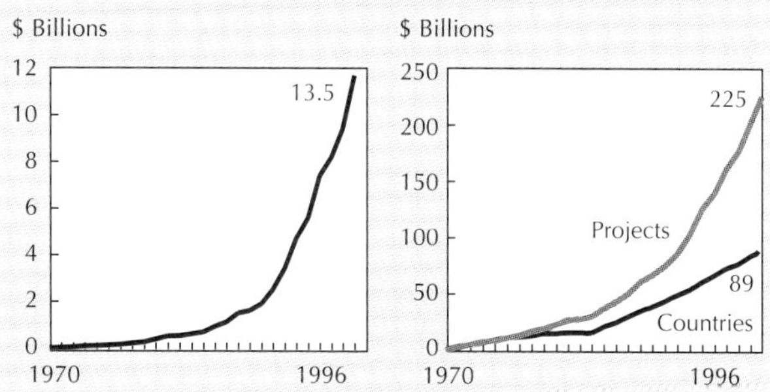

FIGURE 2.2

At the end of FY96, there were 154 active HNP projects in 82 countries with total commitments of US$9.2 billion (1996 prices), and 94 completed projects (see Annex G for map of Active and Future Bank/IDA Financed HNP Projects). About 48 percent of Bank financing from FY94 to FY96 in HNP was IDA credits, targeted to poor countries. Total overseas development assistance to HNP for the period from 1985 through 1993 was about US$2 billion annually in 1996 prices (excluding Bank loans).

Although the HNP portfolio value has expanded rapidly during the past 10 years, there is considerable variation from year to year. FY96 was a record high, with US$2.4 billion in new commitments, compared with approximately US$1.1 billion in FY95 and US$0.9 billion in FY97. The marked increase in FY96 was caused by the approval of five large loans, ranging from US$270 to US$350 million, compared the US$50-60 million average loan size per HNP project and US$80 million Bank average.

Based on the planned pipeline, there will be continued growth in the HNP sector during FY98-FY00, with an expected annual lending of over US$1.5 billion and approximately 22 new projects per year, after discounting by 40 percent for the usual loan drop rate (see Annex E). Disbursements have followed these trends, growing five-fold from US$318 million in FY92 to US$1.5 billion in FY97. The growing portfolio will yield anticipated annual disbursements well above the US$1 billion mark during the next three years.

There are important regional differences in the HNP portfolio (see Annex G for map of Bank regions). The Latin American and Caribbean (LAC) and SAS regions are the biggest users of HNP financing. India is by far the Bank's biggest HNP client. The entry of the ECA region in the early 1990s led to a further rise in total Bank commitments. New approaches are needed to prevent lending in some regions from falling, as countries such as China become ineligible for IDA credits.

Bank Performance in the HNP Sector

Early Bank policy advice, lending, and credits to the HNP sector focused mainly on helping countries strengthen their basic health, nutrition, and population programs. The benefits of interventions in the HNP sector often appear years after specific activities have occurred, and factors outside the sector influence outcomes. It has therefore been difficult to attribute improvements in health status, nutrition, and fertility that have occurred during the past 20 years directly to policy advice and investments made by the Bank.

Early Bank involvement in the HNP sector appears to have been most successful in focusing on capital investment needs, developing infrastructure, and providing supply inputs. Modest success was also achieved in geographic targeting and addressing certain diseases of the poor, partly because policy advice and credits provided under IDA were automatically directed towards poorer countries. This approach was consistent with national HNP policies and a broad international consensus that increasing access to basic services would automatically help improve outcomes.

Unfortunately, capital investments and the supply of inputs are only part of the story. Demand is also an important factor, because goods must be consumed and services used to be effective. People's perceptions about quality and effectiveness of care, the attitudes of health care providers, and the availability of essential consumables such as drugs, have a dramatic impact on utilization. And carelessness in program management and execution, such as a momentary break in a vaccination cold-chain or lack of judgment on when to refer complicated obstetrical cases, can make entire programs ineffective. These factors, which are highly influenced by the availability of adequate recurrent financing, did not receive sufficient attention during the Bank's early involvement in HNP.

Furthermore, reviews by the Operations Evaluation Development (OED) of 120 ongoing projects between FY70 and FY95, and other assessments, have indicated that—although inputs are important to the functioning of basic programs—an input-oriented approach does not achieve the institutional, management, and systemic changes needed to sustain impact over the long run.

First, only 17 percent of completed HNP projects were classified as contributing substantially to institutional development. Several factors seemed to be responsible for this observation: poorly specified institutional development objectives; lack of country commitment; lack of borrower ownership especially in rural areas; inadequate planning and management capacity; inadequate incentives, regulations, information, and communication strategies; poor involvement of non-governmental partners; and lack of attention to monitoring and evaluation. Unrealistic project objectives, complex designs, lack of continuity, and inadequate supervision were other contributing factors.

Second, only 44 percent of completed HNP projects are rated by OED as likely to be sustainable. Poor quality of economic and institutional analysis during project preparation contributed to this failure. This included: inattention to country macro-economic factors; underestimates of recurrent costs implications and insufficient funding to operate constructed facilities; overly optimistic economic benefit assumptions; and poor treatment of intersectoral issues such as civil service, labor market, food subsidy, and tobacco, alcohol, and food taxation policies.

Third, there was often a lack of continuity between the Bank's sectoral policy recommendations and the design of HNP projects. It is instructive to note that, although an increasing number of ongoing projects examine non-governmental roles, none of the 68 completed HNP projects included financing for privately-owned facilities or activities. Furthermore, health systems performance issues were dealt with mainly through public sector interventions, with little attention to the substitution effect and crowding out of private providers. Private sector regulatory and quality control issues were rarely addressed, and few projects have focused specifically on resource mobilization issues.

Finally, recent OED reviews of 68 Project Completion Reports indicate that only 59 percent of these projects had satisfactory ratings, compared with 81 percent in education and 58 percent Bank-wide. Few of these projects provided objective documentation of the impact of project investments on health, fertility, or nutrition outcomes. Since attribution of impact to specific project activities is difficult, input/process/output variables were usually tracked rather than outcomes.

Recently, these observations led the Bank to focus more on systemic reforms, both in the case of broad health systems/financing reforms and in the case of more targeted interventions. Since few of these recent projects have been completed, it is too early to evaluate their success. Based on the FY96 Annual Reviews of Portfolio Performance, the newer HNP projects have kept pace with the 80 percent Bank-wide average in terms of success in development objectives and implementation progress. Causes for concern include the number of projects at risk, the tendency for ratings to deteriorate as the portfolio matures, and the failure of the current peer review system to prevent these problems. Furthermore, there was a significant drop in the resources per project allocated to supervision activities between FY94 and FY96. With the recent increase in attention to quality enhancement and assurance, this trend has reversed itself in FY97 (see Annex E for a more detailed analysis).

In addition to this assessment of the performance of specific investment projects, it is useful to recall that by the end of FY96, more than 100 of the Bank's adjustment operations had some health, nutrition, and/or population content. These have tried to address difficult inter-sectoral and systemic issues such as targeting of the poor, civil service reform, sustainable rural development, decentralization, food policies, protection of social expenditure, cost containment, and tax policy. A thorough assessment of the HNP impact of these projects still needs to be undertaken.

Learning From Experience

Achieving better results requires that the lessons learned through recent reviews of the portfolio by the Quality Assurance Group, the OED, and others be used to improve both the existing portfolio and the quality of new projects. In the past, the lessons learned were often not systematically applied when restructuring old projects or designing new operations. Staff skills-mix and staff-lending ratios also did not keep abreast of portfolio growth and changing priorities.

In the case of the existing portfolio, the *Project at Risk* concept has been developed to provide insights that are not apparent from an analysis of implementation and development objective ratings alone. Some 44 percent of the HNP portfolio was rated "at risk" in early 1997, compared with 30 percent in mid-1996, indicating the importance of an ongoing analysis of this type. Sector managers are now considering how to restructure or cancel some of the projects plagued by: problems of civil unrest or refugee dislocation; slow and uneven implementation in federated states and other decentralized settings; institutional capacity problems in the face of complex project design; and problems relating to procurement, disbursement, and local counterpart funds.

Many of the relevant lessons have been highlighted in past analyses and a working paper on quality assurance (see Box for summary). Few of the recommendations require changes in current policies or procedures, but most require affirmative action.

The past decade may be seen as one of rapid growth and learning in HNP. In the 1980s, US$35 was lent per dollar spent (Bank administrative budget plus consultant trust funds), compared with more than US$60 in FY96 and US$30 in Bank-wide averages. Trust funds—especially Japanese Trust Funds—added over a third to the administrative budget for HNP. This trend is not sustainable. The time is now for action to consolidate the portfolio, to build on previous experience, to avoid past mistakes, and to renew commitment to HNP. Chapter III presents strategies for achieving these goals.

Recommendations for Getting Results in HNP

Ensure quality during project preparation

- **participatory approaches** to encourage client, beneficiary, and stakeholder ownership
- **sectoral analysis** to secure solid knowledge about the issues and options being addressed, linking these to the macro- context of the country in question
- **economic analysis** to inform choices among options, taking into account their costs and impacts
- **institutional analysis** to ensure a realistic assessment of policymaking and implementation capacity
- **sustainability analysis** to assess financial viability, risks, and alternatives (including exit strategies)
- **monitoring and evaluation** to keep projects on track and to draw lessons from experience

Adapt lending policies and procedures to client needs

- test out project ideas on a small scale (**pilot operations**), to learn and incorporate lessons of experience
- use **a process rather than a blueprint approach** for health reform projects
- use **a wider range of instruments**
- accommodate the **highly decentralized nature of the social sectors**
- modify the financing of **recurrent costs**
- extend innovations in **procurement** rules to social sector operations and be more flexible in their application.

Develop and support staff

- build staff capacity through **expanded training, improved incentives, and recruitment of the best**
- strengthen the **professional network and knowledge-sharing system** and **reward excellence**
- familiarize others with HNP sector issues, especially **country managers and procurement advisors**

CHAPTER III

Into the 21st Century: Renewed Commitment and Focus

Sharpening Strategic Directions

The Bank's strategic direction in the HNP sector will continue to evolve in a dynamic way based on international best practice. The complexities of the HNP sector and changing approaches to health, nutrition, and population problems generally do not lend themselves to policy prescriptions. Instead, the policy advice and financial support provided by the Bank will continue to be guided by country-specific approaches to the three major HNP development priorities outlined in Chapter I and described in more detail below.

> ***HNP Priority One:* To work with countries to improve the health, nutrition, and population outcomes of the world's poor, and to protect the population from the impoverishing effects of illness, malnutrition, and high fertility.**

This strategy requires greater emphasis on designing and monitoring programs that improve outcomes for the poor. A variety of approaches is needed to adapt this strategy to specific country and local settings, especially in low-income countries where most of the rural population is often living below the poverty line, and in middle-income countries with significant pockets of residual poverty. The Bank will encourage the selective use of the targeting mechanisms described in Chapter I. It will emphasize the needs of the most vulnerable, such as women and children, and the areas where scarce public resources will have the greatest impact, such as preventive public health activities with large externalities. The latter would include protecting the poor against high risk behavior such as smoking and the consumption of alcohol and unhealthy foods.

High fertility remains a major health and social challenge in low-income countries. The Bank will continue to emphasize the need for effective population and nutrition policies to improve family planning and other reproductive health services that help to increase the demand for smaller family size, and to reduce unwanted fertility. Likewise, in low-income countries, making food more affordable, increasing the efficiency of food markets, and providing nutrition safety nets can have a significant impact on health that reaches beyond what can be achieved through improvement in health services.

Addressing these problems often requires a broad range of social policies that improve and expand the life choices available to the poor, especially girls and women, including greater gender equality in education and improvements in the status of women. Where women leave home to earn money in the daytime, good childcare can be as critical to improving child health as health services, if associated with appropriate nutrition and preventive programs (e.g. immunization and dental care). Addressing such problems may also require paying more attention to traditional values and attitudes, such as female patients not wanting to be treated by male doctors or low-income rural populations not feeling comfortable seeking care in alienating institutional settings.

Due to transportation costs and direct loss of income, the poor often fail to seek care if they have to travel far only to receive low quality services, even when such care is highly subsidized. The Bank will emphasize the need to stimulate appropriate demand in these settings, including that of traditional family units.

In very low-income countries, the international donor community must also strive to replace piecemeal assistance with more coordinated sector-wide approaches. The central objectives will be to enhance technical, managerial, and political capacity, reduce donor dependence over time, and secure minimum levels of essential health, nutrition, and family planning services, even if these are at lower levels than is desirable and feasible in higher income countries. In some countries, such action is urgently needed to bridge the financing gap while medium- to long-term economic growth objectives are pursued.

The Bank can also make a significant contribution to the health of the poor at the inter-country and regional level. The Onchocerciasis Control Program (river blindness), the African Population Advisory Committee, and the *Better Health in Africa* Expert Panel are helping to adapt international initiatives to African realities and to empower African leaders to take charge of HNP challenges. Whether in disease control (e.g. malaria), or reducing micro-nutrient deficiency (e.g. salt iodization), inter-country action has significant potential to help some of the world's poorest countries.

Finally, the Bank will encourage governments to address often-neglected multi-sectoral issues such as food and agricultural policies, environment, water supply, sanitation, and transportation that often have an indirect impact on health. In particular, the Bank will encourage governments to introduce aggressive policies to counter the adverse health effects of mass marketing and inappropriate use of tobacco products and alcohol.

To implement this strategy, the Bank needs to work more closely not only with ministries of health, but also with other ministries and stakeholders that address poverty and population issues as well as basic infrastructure and rural community issues. Within the Bank, closer links will be established between the Human Development (HD) Network, the Poverty Reduction and Economic Management (PREM) Network, and the Environment and Socially Sustainable Development (ESSD) Network to ensure that health, nutrition, and population programs designed to assist the poor are an integral part of broader poverty alleviation and rural development strategies.

***HNP Priority Two:* To work with countries to enhance the performance of health care systems by promoting equitable access and use of population-based preventive and curative HNP services that are affordable, effective, well managed, of good quality, and responsive to client needs.**

Sector-wide reforms are often needed in countries with serious systemic HNP sector problems. Although there will be some overlap, the approach emphasized in low-income countries will often differ from that recommended in middle-income countries. In low-income countries, where private sector activities often dominate (see Annex A for a listing of countries with more than 70 percent of health care expenditure in the private sector), governments will be encouraged to focus their attention on the provision of: services with large externalities (preventive public health services); essential clinical services for the poor; and more effective regulations for the private sector. They will also be encouraged to strengthen their management capacity, support R&D and medical education, and secure sustainable financing (see HNP priority three), quality assurance, and client satisfication.

In some low-income countries and many middle-income countries, where public sector activities dominate (see Annex A for a listing of countries with more than 70 percent of health care expenditure in the public sector), governments will be encouraged to promote greater diversity in service delivery systems by providing funding for civil society and non-governmental providers on a competitive basis, instead of limiting public funds to public facilities. In many of these instances, rebalancing the public-private interface will be preferable to an outright privatization of social assets. Quasi-market mechanisms, such as vouchers, competitive contracting-out, and the increased use of client feedback, can both improve public sector performance and encourage quality participation by the private sector.

Where institutional capacity for financing and regulation is weak, a gradual approach emphasizing decentralization and internal markets is better than actively transferring ownership of public facilities, with all its attendant employment and political consequences. In stronger institutional settings—when there is an appropriate and effective regulatory environment—a more active participation by non governmental providers can be encouraged.

Governments need to become more effective in policymaking, sectoral management, outcome evaluation, and regulation. Government and non-governmental actors (professional associations, consumer groups, and academic institutions) will be encouraged to generate knowledge about improving access, the effectiveness of specific interventions, and efficiency in managing services, controlling quality, and responding to client needs. Effective incentives and provider payment mechanisms can make a significant contribution to improving the performance of health systems.

To implement this strategy, the Bank needs to work closely not only with ministries of health, but also with ministries of finance, privatization, and planning. Within the Bank, closer links will be established with the IFC and the Finance, Private Sector, and Infrastructure (FPSI) Network to build on lessons learned about divestiture of social assets and to facilitate the flow of finance to non-governmental recipients.

> ***HNP Priority Three:* To work with countries in securing sustainable health care financing by mobilizing adequate levels of resources, establishing broad-based risk pooling mechanisms, and maintaining effective control over public and private expenditure.**

The experience of most low- and middle-income countries, as well as all OECD countries, suggests that governments must play a major role in health care financing through regulations, mandates, and direct subsidies. Although considerable private resources may be available, these resources are often wasted on ineffective care without effective government policies.

Based on this experience, the Bank needs to become more active in helping countries to secure sustainable recurrent financing for health, nutrition, and population programs, rather than in providing resources just for capital investments. The mix of taxation instruments (social insurance and general revenues) and copayments needs to be tailored to each country. In low-income countries, significant efforts are needed to complement public resources with non-governmental community-based financing and international assistance (see Annex A for list of low-income countries that fail to mobilize the minimal levels of financing needed to pay for essential services for the poor). At middle- and higher-income levels, taxation instruments become a more efficient way to mobilize financial resources and expand risk pooling. Special attention will be given to the associated fiscal and labor market implications (see Annex A for list of high-spending countries where fiscal implications may be a potential concern).

Governments will also be encouraged to maintain effective expenditure control and to ensure that the HNP budget envelope is used on effective and quality care that benefits those who need it most.

Experience has shown that when middle-income countries expand coverage and begin to use a fuller range of financing instruments, strong government action is needed to prevent an expenditure explosion in the health sector such as occurred in Argentina, the Czech Republic, Jordan, and South Africa. The Bank will take active steps to learn more about how to assist these countries.

To implement this strategy, the Bank needs to work closely with ministries of finance and ministries of social security as principal counterparts in addition to ministries of health. Within the Bank, the HNP Family will work closely with the Poverty Reduction and Economic Management (PREM) Network in this work.

Achieving Greater Impact

The major expansion of the Bank's work in HNP is now about a decade old. The rapid growth has led to uneven quality, fragmentation of emphasis, and substantial concerns about impact and effectiveness. To implement the strategy set out in this document, maximize the impact of investments, and ensure that clients receive the best possible service, the Bank needs to follow four principles: emphasize strategic policy direction; underpin lending with analysis and research; increase selectivity; and improve client services. These are explained in more detail below.

Emphasizing Strategic Policy Directions

HNP strategies have a development timeframe of 10 to 15 years, which exceeds the life cycle of most projects (five to eight years), individual staff assignments (three to five years), and ministers' terms in office (one to four years). Given this constraint, it is critical that the country-specific HNP strategies presented in each CAS—as well as the Bank's policy advice, lending, and research agenda—focus explicitly on both medium-term objectives and shorter-term activities consistent with the three HNP priority areas described above.

The CAS will be used as a key instrument for delivering the Bank's message about HNP priorities during high-level country dialogue. HNP staff will work more closely with country teams on the CAS in those countries that have been identified as having particularly serious systemic problems in the HNP sector (see Annex A for country rankings under each of the three HNP priority areas). HNP staff will also work more closely with the education and social protection sectors to develop quantitative measures for human capital formation and labor productivity, which could be included in the analytical framework that is routinely used to underpin CAS recommendations. Management will selectively monitor progress made in improving outcomes, health systems performance, and health financing indicators in countries that have been identified as being at greatest risk.

Underpinning Lending with Analysis and Research

As the Bank continues to shift from a focus on physical inputs and outputs to a greater emphasis on outcome and process, it needs to experiment and learn. This can best be accomplished through rigorous design, supervision, and evaluation of pilot projects, and by placing greater emphasis on the design and supervision of the research components of investment projects.

Areas for increased attention include: (a) understanding more fully individual and household responses to prices, quality, access, public health policies, specific interventions, the public/private interface, and various aspects of the health production function; (b) encouraging individuals and households to take more responsibility for their own health and to participate in decision making; (c) exploring the factors that influence performance of health systems such as the political economy of reforms, governance, and institutional dimensions; (d) learning more about how to secure sustainable health care financing and broad risk pooling, and how to use the results from health expenditure reviews (public and private) to set sectoral priorities (resource allocation decisions and cost containment); and, (e) drawing out the experience from health sector reforms across countries to clarify the relationships between intersectoral policies, health system performance, financing, and outcomes.

Fulfilling this agenda requires a reversal of recent cutbacks in sectoral analysis, an increase in the budget for HNP research in line with the HNP portfolio size, and a greater allocation of resources to help design and implement innovative projects. In the future, the HNP Family of the HD Network will ensure that staff make more effective use of lessons learned from past experience (positive and negative).

Increasing Selectivity

The Bank cannot do everything well. Difficult choices must be made about where to intervene and where to support other organizations or the private sector. The Bank will continue to work closely with its partner organizations, such as WHO, in defining a clearer division of labor to promote greater complementarity and to avoid wasteful duplication. Product selectivity can be improved by screening prospective projects based on: (a) country needs in the three HNP priority areas; (b) an objective assessment of the potential benefits—emphasizing activities that are associated with large externalities—and associated political, institutional, and economic risks; and (c) commitment to significant reform.

Selectivity in terms of countries needs to be considered carefully. One way for the Bank to maximize its impact on the poor is to concentrate effort and resources on the cluster of countries in which most of the poor live (see Annex A for low-income country groupings).

Selectivity based on the degree to which policy dialogue and project activities influence the allocation of existing recurrent expenditure is another way for the Bank to leverage its financing. Annual IDA resources play a significant role in total health sector financing in smaller poor countries (16.4 percent in Sub-Saharan Africa and 13.1 percent in South Asia, excluding India) but not in larger ones (0.5 percent in China and 0.7 percent in India). Annual IBRD assistance to middle-income countries is similarly insignificant (0.6 percent in Jordan, 0.4 percent in Poland, 0.3 percent in Argentina, and 0.2 percent in Mexico).

Finally, the CASs could provide a powerful tool for increasing selectivity by focusing on HNP issues that require broad systemic and multi-sectoral interventions, where the Bank has the greatest comparative advantage.

Improving Client Services

The quality of services offered by the Bank to clients in the HNP sector can be improved in several ways. First, the Bank will strengthen its HNP knowledge base. This will include establishing: (a) health, nutrition, and population help desks; (b) an on-line database of policy papers, best practice papers, electronic forums, terms-of-reference, profiles of staff and consultants, and links to external resources; (c) a Bank database on health expenditure trends and a clearinghouse function for other HNP data; and (d) a knowledge base on various other aspects of HNP systems such as demand and utilization patterns, behavior of providers, and health care markets. The Bank will also keep up with global best practice and developments in the HNP sector.

Second, more time and effort will be spent learning about portfolio performance and applying the lessons learned more systematically, both during project design and implementation. This requires learning more about what constitutes good project design by applying the available tools of sectoral, economic, institutional, and risk analysis. More time is also needed to pilot new approaches such as broad sector reforms and public/private partnerships. Projects that clearly fail to meet their development objectives will be restructured, or canceled if they fail to improve after a reasonable time. Finally, an effort will be made to learn more about how to influence external factors, such as political commitment from one administration to another, and how to deal with the institutional resistance when stakeholder interests are threatened by reform proposals.

Third, a more flexible and broad range of lending instruments will be tested. This includes greater use of sector-wide approaches and adjustment loans to support systemic reforms, and the use of the new micro-, mini- and adaptable investment loans once they become available. The use of smaller and innovative free-standing loans will avoid adding complex sub-components to standard projects. A Bank study has already begun to explore the use of simpler and more flexible procurement and processing procedures.

Given the importance of good assessments of client needs and communication strategies to health, nutrition, and population outcomes, user satisfaction surveys will be initiated and used to inform future project designs.

Monitoring Development Impact

The ultimate objective of work in the HNP sector is to improve health, nutrition, and population outcomes, health systems performance, and health care financing. The Bank needs to take steps to improve its own and borrower capacity to monitor and evaluate progress in achieving these objectives.

The tables in Annex A summarize key health, nutrition, and population issues for the world, for low-, middle- and high-income countries, and for the Bank's regions. They also measure performance under the three different HNP priority areas based on general economic and other human development determinants, indicators of health, nutrition, and population status, health systems and health financing indicators, and data pointing to future challenges in the HNP sector.

The indicators for performance of health systems are weak. The Bank will work with other international organizations and client countries to develop more effective indicators, introduce incentives to encourage their use (recognition, rewards, and reviews), and include monitoring and evaluation components as integral parts of project designs. The future pipeline, and restructuring of the current portfolio, will be guided by the likely impact on these indicators.

Empowering Staff

The underpinnings for improved staff development and management have already been initiated by the recent establishment of an HD Network and Council, the HNP Family and Sector Board, and the Regional Sector Heads (see Figure D.2 in Annex D). Key staffing issues relating to the Bank's capacity to meet its objectives in the HNP sector include: skills mix, number of staff, and deployment.

First, recruitment, staff training opportunities, and HNP sector professional standards will be adjusted to reflect the sharpened policy directions. Priority is being placed on the broad skills needed to deal with a wider range of products and to address more effectively the three HNP priority areas. Special emphasis will be given to staff who have practical experience in the HNP sector, are able to work with complex policy issues, and understand the political economy of reform processes.

Second, the Bank needs to assure staffing in the HNP sector reflects the size and growth of the HNP portfolio. Lending to the HNP sector during the past decade has grown more rapidly than staff. HNP staff numbers increased by 86 percent between FY86 and FY96, whereas lending grew by 272 percent. More recently, the average annual rate of growth of HNP sector staff of 6 percent has continued to lag behind the expected 13 percent annual increase in lending. The new Network structure is expected to improve the efficiency of staff in the sector. The issue of assuring adequate staffin in the sector is a management priority.

Finally, the Bank needs to explore two approaches to bringing staff closer to clients. One approach, inspired by the experience of the India resident mission, is to have a senior Bank specialist oversee the work of a group of locally-hired staff within a single country. Another approach is to coordinate the staff in several resident missions through a regional hub, such as the human development team in the Budapest resident mission. Improved communications links between headquarters staff, field staff, and clients help to bridge the gap in cases where direct contacts are not possible.

In the case of training activities, the HNP Family of the HD Network will: link training to the three strategic directions in the HNP sector; include both Bank staff and clients; increase opportunities for resident mission staff; and extend the target audience to sectors outside HNP. Improving management skills of HNP staff will be given particularly high priority.

Strengthening Partnerships

To meet the development challenges of the 21st century, the Bank needs to strengthen its partnerships with clients, civil society, stakeholders, and other agencies. WHO and the Bank have made great progress over the past two years in clarifying their comparative advantages and optimizing their collaboration in the interests of client countries. Two key forms of collaboration have been agreed upon: (a) country-level collaboration in which WHO technical expertise is mobilized to improve the design, supervision, and evaluation of Bank-supported projects; and (b) global collaboration in which WHO and the Bank join forces to advance international understanding of health, nutrition, and population issues. Similar efforts are being made with UNAIDS, UNFPA, UNICEF, and other agencies.

The Bank's collaboration with other agencies on international research and development (R&D) will be strengthened. First, the Bank will continue to support the newly-established Global Forum on Health Research using funds from the Special Grants Program. The Forum provides a mechanism for focusing R&D resources more tightly on priority subjects, including health policy research, low-cost management of non-communicable diseases, and slowing the spread of drug-resistant microbes. Second, the continuation of grant financing for priority international initiatives that improve and share knowledge in the fields of nutrition and reproductive health will be encouraged. Third, in partnership with the Forum, the Bank will collaborate with the pharmaceutical, vaccine, and biotechnology industries to strengthen the R&D pipeline for products needed by poor people in low-income countries—such as new drugs for drug resistant malaria, a better vaccine for tuberculosis, and improved diagnostics for sexually transmitted diseases. Finally the Bank will seek ways to extend its support for the International AIDS Vaccine Initiative (IAVI), UNAIDS, and the private sector in the newly heightened search for an AIDS vaccine.

An effort will also be made to replicate in other areas the Bank's successful partnership with other organizations in river blindness control and to support other international health, nutrition, and population initiatives with potentially large externalities. Likely candidates include collaboration with African governments and others in a major effort to control the malaria epidemic on that continent, and work with WHO and others to combat the pandemic of tuberculosis and to promote integrated management of childhood illness.

From Vision to Action

Implementation of the HNP strategy will be linked closely with the Bank's new Strategic Compact. In close consultation with staff at the regional level, the HNP Sector Board will translate the objectives and broad action plan outlined in the Strategy Matrix in Annex F into clear performance benchmarks against which the Bank will be judged by the time of the next HNP Sector Strategy Paper.

Through such action, the Bank expects to enhance its role in the global effort to improve human development during the first decade of the 21st century. The Bank will continue to inform and influence the terms of the global health policy debate and to strengthen partnerships with its clients and fellow agencies.

ANNEX A

HNP Sector At A Glance: Global, Regional, and Country Profiles

Background

The indicators shown in the following tables include general economic and other human development determinants, indicators of health, nutrition, and population status, health finance and health systems indicators, and future challenges in the health sector. Tables include: (a) regional ranking of high risk countries by HNP indicators, (b) global ranking of countries by HNP indicators, and (c) *HNP At a Glance* tables for the world, for high income countries, for six regions, and for individual countries.

Regional and Global Ranking by HNP Indicators

Table A.1 and A.2 show countries with high health risks. The first table shows the ranking of low- and middle-income countries on eight key HNP determinants and outcomes. This table shows that some countries and some regions rank consistently high in terms of poor HNP outcomes and risks.

The second table shows ten countries per region that have poor outcomes on HNP indicators or determinants, as defined in the table. In some regions for some of the indicators, there are fewer than ten countries 'at risk'; in other regions the number of countries exceeds ten, but only ten are shown in the order of highest risk or poorest outcomes first.

HNP At a Glance: World

Table A.3 shows the level of indicators by region for each of the following broad categories:

- Key Economic Indicators
- Average Annual Growth
- Human Development Determinants
- Health Indicators
- Nutrition Indicators
- Reproductive Health Indicators
- Future Challenges
- Health Services Indicators
- Health Finance Indicators

HNP At A Glance: High Income and Regions

Table A.4 covers a number of countries in each region selected on the basis of: (a) largest population; (b) poverty-related HNP indicators; (c) selected indicators for health systems performance; and (d) selected indicators for health expenditure. Table A.4 also shows averages for low- and middle-income countries and for each region as a whole. Table A.5 covers at-risk countries among high-income countries.

Largest Population

The country with the largest population is also the country with the largest HNP portfolio in all regions except

MNA. The HNP indicators of these countries have the largest impact on the regional averages that are population weighted.

Indicators of Poverty and HNP Outcomes

Four poverty-related indicators are used as criteria to select countries:

Lowest per capita income in the region. A strong association between income and health status is evident, with the poorest country showing below-average performance on most HNP status indicators in all regions.

Highest under-5 mortality rate (or next highest, if this duplicates the country with the lowest income). Under-5 mortality captures the impact of poverty on health better than infant mortality or other mortality indicators. It measures the combined effect of nutrition, access to immunization and curative health services, and local conditions. High under-5 mortality has a large impact on overall life expectancy; no country with an under-5 mortality rate of over 50 has a life expectancy of 70 or above.

Highest child malnutrition prevalence (or next highest, if this duplicates the country with the lowest income). High child malnutrition is associated with poor performance on several other health indicators, as well as with other child development aspects. This indicator has a strong regional association: it is high in most countries in the South Asia and East Asia and Pacific regions.

Highest total fertility (or next highest, if this duplicates the country with the lowest income). Countries with high fertility usually have high population growth rates, large proportions of young people, and often high adolescent fertility rates. Maternal mortality is also associated with high fertility, especially when considered as the life-time risk of dying from pregnancy-related causes. High fertility is frequently found in poor households, and poverty and high fertility are mutually reinforcing.

Selected Indicators of Health Care Coverage

The following two indicators address two aspects of health systems. Access to health services shows the potential of health systems to improve health status. Immunization rates show the realized performance of the health system.

Lowest measles immunization rate. High measles immunization rates have been achieved in many countries in the developing world, averaging about 76 percent in the early 1990s. A low level of immunization is an indication of a failing health delivery system.

Lowest access to health services (or next lowest, if there is a duplication in previous indicator). The percent of the population within one hour's walk or travel to health service providers measures the availability of health services to the population.

Selected Indicators of Health Expenditure

The percent of GDP spent on health is of interest both as a determinant of health outcomes and equity, and as an indicator of efficiency and fiscal burdens. The following indicators were selected to illustrate these issues:

Low public expenditure (as percent of GDP) on health care. Countries with very low public expenditures are usually the poorest performers on a range of health status indicators. Concern is warranted if public expenditure is less than 2 percent of GDP or total expenditure is less than 3 percent of GDP. Such countries are probably not allocating a sufficient share of national resources to providing poor populations and other vulnerable groups with protection against illness.

High total expenditure (as percent of GDP) on health care. There are no firm guidelines on what constitutes too much expenditure on health care. However, in some countries, the share of national product and public resources spent on health care are greater than expenditure on education and other social programs that also contribute significantly to poverty reduction, economic growth, and overall well-being. Fiscal concern is warranted in low- and middle-income countries if total health spending is greater than 7 percent of GDP. In some of these countries, the extensive use of general revenues and payroll-based taxes in the formal employment sector probably has some negative implications for labor costs, commodity prices, international competitiveness, and overall tax compliance.

HNP At a Glance: Countries

Table A.6 provides data for over 200 countries using the same indicators as shown in the regional tables, A.4 and A.5.

Definitions

Access to health services. The percent of the population covered for treatment of common diseases and injuries, including availability of essential drugs, within one hour's walk or travel. Source: World Bank, World Development Indicators, 1997, based on and supplemented with data collected by WHO and UNICEF.

Access to safe water. The share of the population with reasonable access to an adequate amount of safe water (including treated surface water and untreated but uncontaminated well and spring water). Source: World Bank, World Development Indicators, 1997, based on and supplemented with data collected by WHO and UNICEF.

Adolescent fertility rate. This measures the fertility rate for women under age 20, shown per 1000 women under age 20. These are estimates and projections based on Demographic and Health Surveys, national estimates, and other sources of age-specific fertility rates. For some countries that lack age-specific fertility schedules, the figures are based on models.

Adult HIV/AIDS prevalence. This measures the percentage of those over age 15 who are HIV positive. Source: UNAIDS, based on blood screening of pregnant women, blood donors, and the general population.

Adult mortality rate. The probability of dying between ages 15 and 60 based on prevailing mortality rates. These are World Bank estimates based on model life tables selected on the basis of overall life expectancy and infant and under-5 mortality. For countries with vital registration-based life tables, a close fit between these model-based estimates and the life table values has been found. However, such agreement cannot be assumed for all countries, and the data presented here should be interpreted as indicative of the level of adult mortality rather than as precise estimates.

Anemia—iron deficiency. This is defined as hemoglobin levels less than 11 grams per deciliter among pregnant women. Source: WHO data and Micronutrients Initiative.

Child malnutrition rate. Prevalence of malnutrition is measured as the percentage of children under age five whose weight for age is less than minus two standard deviations from the median of the reference population. The data are mostly from WHO, supplemented with data from UNICEF and the Administrative Coordination Committee/Subcommittee on Nutrition.

External debt. This represents the discounted present value of future debt service payments, including private, public, and publicly guaranteed short-term and long-term debt. The discount rate reflects market lending rates for the currency in which the loan is denominated.

Gini coefficient. This index measures the extent to which the distribution of income among individuals or households deviates from a perfectly equal distribution. A Gini index of zero represents perfect equality while an index of 100 percent implies perfect inequality. Source: World Bank, World Development Indicators, 1997, based on household surveys conducted during the period 1990 to 1995.

Gross domestic investment. This consists of outlays on additions to fixed assets of the economy, plus net changes in the level of inventories. Data for developing countries are collected from national statistical organizations and central banks by World Bank staff. Data for industrial countries are from OECD data files.

GDP (at purchasers' prices). This is the sum of the gross value added by all resident and nonresident producers in the economy, plus any taxes and minus any subsidies not included in the value of the products. It is calculated without making deductions for depreciation of fabricated assets or for depletion and degradation of natural resources. Data for developing countries are collected from national statistical offices and central banks by World Bank staff. Data for industrial countries come from OECD data files.

GNP per capita, (US dollars). From World Development Indicators, 1997. GNP per capita is derived from GNP converted to US dollars (using the World Bank Atlas method) divided by the midyear population.

Gross secondary enrollment ratio. The ratio of total enrollment, regardless of age, to the population of the age group that officially corresponds to the total level of education. Source: World Bank, World Development Indicators, 1997, based on the 1995 Statistical Yearbook from the United Nations Educational, Scientific, and Cultural Organization (UNESCO).

Health expenditure (private). This includes spending on health from the following sources: direct household expenditure (out-of-pocket), private insurance, charitable donations, and direct service payments by private corporations. Data are from World Bank, PAHO, IMF, and other studies.

Health expenditure (public). This consists of spending from the following sources: government (local and central) budgets, external borrowings and grants, and social (or compulsory) health insurance funds. All external assistance, including donations from international NGOs, is included under the public expenditure category. Public health expenditure is reflected in US dollars, PPP exchange rate, and as a percent of GDP. Data are from World Bank, PAHO, IMF, and other studies.

Health expenditure (total). This includes outlays for the provision of health services (preventive and curative), population activities, nutrition activities, and emergency aid designated for health. It does not include water and sanitation. Figures are for actual year from which most recent data is available. Total health expenditure includes both public and private health expenditures and is reflected in US dollars, PPP exxchange rate, and as a percent of GDP. Data are from World Bank, PAHO, IMF, and other studies.

Immunization of children under 12 months for measles, DPT. The percentage of children under 12 months immunized against measles (one dose of vaccine) and DPT (diphtheria, pertussis, and tetanus; at least two of three doses of vaccine). Source: World Bank, World Development Indicators, 1997, based on and supplemented with data collected by WHO and UNICEF.

Infant mortality rate. The number of deaths of infants under age one per 1,000 births. These are based on country statistical offices, censuses and surveys, World Bank sector studies, and—especially for countries without reliable data—the UN Population Division's estimates. For many developing countries without reliable vital registration, indirect estimates from demographic surveys are used.

In-patient hospital beds. This measure includes beds available in public and private, general, and specialized hospitals and rehabilitation centers. Hospitals are establishments permanently staffed by at least one physician. Data are from government statistical yearbooks, World Bank, OECD, and WHO.

Life expectancy at birth. The average number of years a newborn will live based on prevailing mortality rates. Note that by definition these are based on period life tables, and may not apply to any cohort for which mortality conditions may be different in subsequent years. The sources for the data include the UN Population Division, national statistical offices, and World Bank estimates and projections from surveys and censuses. For most countries, 1995 life expectancy estimates are projections based on the trend in the previous decade. HIV/AIDS prevalence data are used to adjust the trend, and account for the declining life expectancy in countries where AIDS mortality is high.

Low birth weight. Defined as children born weighing less than 2,500 grams, with the measurement taken within the first hours of life, before significant postnatal weight loss has occurred. Source: World Bank, World Development Indicators, 1997.

Maternal mortality ratio. This measures the number of deaths to women during pregnancy and childbirth per 100,000 live births in the same year. The estimates are from the Demographic and Health Surveys, national estimates, and, for countries without such data, from a model developed by WHO and UNICEF that is based on fertility and other variables related to maternal mortality. The measurement of maternal mortality is often inaccurate due to underreporting in vital registration, large standard errors in survey-based estimates, and the use of indirect methods that produce estimates for past years. All maternal mortality estimates, but especially the model-based figures, should be seen as indicative.

Obesity prevalence. This measures the percentage of the population with a body mass index of 30 or higher. Data denoted 'a' are for adults, data denoted 'b' are for children. Sources for the data are the FAO and the Demographic and Health Surveys.

Population. Midyear estimates and projections of total de-facto population. Refugees not permanently settled in the country of asylum are excluded from the estimates. Sources of population estimates vary from country to country, and are based on the most recent census, official country estimates, UN Population Division estimates, or on data from other international agencies. Projections are based on the cohort component methodology, in which a baseline age-sex structure is projected with fertility, mortality, and migration schedules. For a detailed description of the methodology and assumptions, see: World Bank, World Population Projections, 1994–95.

Population growth rates. These are average annual rates expressed in percentages, calculated from midyear estimates and projections using an exponential rate of change.

Purchasing Power Parity conversion factor. The number of units of a country's currency required to buy the same amounts of goods and services in the domestic market as a dollar would buy in the United States. Source: World Bank staff estimates.

Physicians. Defined as graduates of any faculty or school of medicine who are working in the country in any medical field (practice, teaching, research). Data are from government statistical yearbooks, World Bank, OECD and WHO.

Smoking prevalence. Percent of males and females over age 15 who smoke tobacco products. Sources are WHO and country surveys for the most recent year.

Total fertility rate. This measures the average number of children born per women entering the childbearing age, if subject to prevailing fertility rates. The sources are the Demographic and Health Surveys, World Fertility Surveys, Contraceptive Prevalence Surveys, other demographic surveys, vital registration, World Bank staff estimates, and the UN Population Division. As with some of the mortality data, estimates of past fertility are frequently based on indirect estimates from survey data.

Tuberculosis incidence. This shows the estimated number of new sputum smear positive (SS+) cases per 100,00 population in Tables A.3 to A.5, and the estimated TB incidence (all forms) in Table A.6. Source: WHO 1997 Global Tuberculosis Control Report.

Under-5 mortality rate. This measures the probability that a newborn will survive to exactly age five, based on prevailing mortality rates, times 1,000. The estimates from 1960 to 1990 are based on a methodology developed by Hill and Yazbeck (1994) using regression analysis. Weighted least-square regression was used in their analysis, assigning weights to each country's data on the basis of the validity of the data. Figures for 1995 are World Bank staff estimates based on published sources such as UNICEF's State of the World's Children 1997 and on projections from the latest available survey, census, and vital registration data.

Urban population. This measures the percentage of a country's total population residing in urban areas. Definitions of urban areas are country specific, and vary considerably among countries. Source: UN Population Division, World Urbanization Prospects, the 1994 Revision.

Unwanted fertility. Unwanted births are defined as those that exceed the number considered ideal by women of reproductive age. This is used to calculate a "total wanted fertility rate", in the same manner that the total fertility rate is calculated. The difference between the total fertility rate and the wanted fertility rate is the unwanted fertility rate. Women who do not report a numerical ideal family size are assumed to want all their births. Source: Demographic and Health Surveys (conducted in the past seven years).

Burden of Disease, Prevalence, and Risk Factors

Burden of disease may be understood as the gap between the health status of a population and some reference of its good health. Measuring the burden is helpful as one tool to rationally prioritize among various health interventions, or to provide a quantitative basis for planning health services. In practice, the burden of disease may be measured by a number of indicators of morbidity and mortality. These include the frequency with which a disease or disability occurs within a population, the death rate, or an index that combines measures of morbidity and mortality, such as disability-adjusted life years (DALYs).

Understanding the epidemiologic characteristics of a disease is useful in understanding how health interventions may work in a population. The burden of disease is a function of a number of epidemiologic characteristics, including frequency, duration, and severity.

$$\text{Burden of Disease} = f\,(\text{frequency, duration, severity})$$

Prevalence may be thought of as the proportion of the population with a given disease at any given point in time.

$$\text{Prevalence} = \frac{\text{number with disease}}{\text{total population size}}$$

The incidence rate of disease represents the number of new cases of a condition in the population within a specified time frame, such as one year. As a measure of the frequency of a disease, incidence reflects the probability or risk of a health event occurring. Prevalence rates are different from incidence rates because they measure the frequency of both new and existing cases of a disease. While prevalence is a measure of disease burden (e.g. the frequency of diabetes in a population), it is not a measure of the risk of getting a disease. The duration of the disease is what links incidence to the prevalence of a disease, commonly expressed as:

$$\text{Prevalence} = \text{Incidence} \times \text{Duration}$$

Risk factors are attributes or exposures that are associated with the probability of a health outcome, such as the occurrence of a disease, its duration, or severity. Some risk factors are known to be causally related to certain health outcomes. For example, contaminated water supplies increase the risk of diarrhea, and smoking increases the incidence of cancers, heart disease, and stroke. Some types of risk factors broadly influence the incidence of disease, but are not immediate causes of illness. These type of determinants include income, education, and social class. Poor population groups generally have a much higher incidence of most diseases than do rich groups. The poor also tend to have higher case fatality rates, one measure of the severity of disease. The case fatality rate is the proportion of people with a specific condition who die within a given time period. Other measures of severity indicate the degree of disability among those surviving with a disease.

The incidence of disease may be reduced by some types of preventive health measures, such as immunizations. The duration of illness, the case fatality rate, and other indicators of severity may be affected by both preventive and curative health services. For example, antibiotics prevent deaths from acute respiratory infection, and low-cost de-worming agents reduce morbidity from intestinal worms. Other types of risk factors also matter, and suggest other points of intervention. For example, malnutrition and vitamin A deficiency increase the case fatality rate of measles. Income, education, and other broad determinants may affect case fatality rates or disease duration, possibly through differences in utilization of health services, healthy behaviors, or exposure to other risk factors. Fatality is, of course, inevitable for all persons and for some diseases despite health services.

Health systems are concerned largely with the health of populations, and aim to decrease incidence by reducing known risk factors, and to increase survival or the quality of life by providing health services or changing behaviors affecting health. Health systems can also affect the broad socioeconomic determinants of good health and illness indirectly, through the relationships between health, productivity, and ability to earn income.

Table A.1 Global Ranking of At-Risk Countries by HNP Indicators, Low- and Middle-Income Countries

	Poverty and HNP Outcome Indicators				*Coverage Indicators*	
	GNP per capita Low ⇨ High	*Under-5 mortality rate* High ⇨ Low	*Under-5 malnutrition* High ⇨ Low	*Fertility rate* High ⇨ Low	*Immunization coverage* Low ⇨ High	*Access to health services* Low ⇨ High
1	Mozambique	Liberia	Bangladesh	Niger	Chad	Central African Rep.
2	Ethiopia	Afghanistan	India	Yemen, Rep.	Niger	Cameroon
3	Tanzania	Sierra Leone	Nepal	Gaza Strip	Angola	Angola
4	Zaire	Guinea-Bissau	Ethiopia	Oman	Haiti	Ghana
5	Burundi	Malawi	Mauritania	Ethiopia	Zaire	Chad
6	Malawi	Guinea	Mozambique	Somalia	Cote d'Ivoire	Mozambique
7	Chad	Somalia	Viet Nam	Angola	Central African Rep.	Niger
8	Rwanda	Gambia, The	Niger	Afghanistan	Sierra Leone	Senegal
9	Sierra Leone	Angola	Eritrea	Mali	Nigeria	Benin
10	Nepal	Rwanda	Afghanistan	Burkina Faso	Eritrea	Indonesia
11	Niger	Chad	Lao PDR	Uganda	Mali	Guinea
12	Burkina Faso	Eritrea	Pakistan	Maldives	Burkina Faso	Haiti
13	Madagascar	Mali	Indonesia	Malawi	Cameroon	Ethiopia
14	Bangladesh	Mozambique	Somalia	Liberia	Gabon	Thailand
15	Uganda	Ethiopia	Maldives	Lao PDR	Congo	Zaire
16	Guinea-Bissau	Equatorial Guinea	Bhutan	Burundi	Mauritania	Guatemala
17	Haiti	Djibouti	Cambodia	Sierra Leone	Papua New Guinea	Cote d'Ivoire
18	Mali	Zambia	Sri Lanka	Guinea	Italy	Morocco
19	Nigeria	Nigeria	Burundi	Togo	Lao PDR	Honduras
20	Yemen, Rep.	Bhutan	Angola	Mozambique	Yemen, Rep.	Madagascar

	Health Expenditure Indicators			
	Public health expenditures/GDP Low ⇨ High	*Total health expenditures/GDP* High ⇨ Low	*Public expenditures > 70% of total* High ⇨ Low	*Private expenditures > 70% of total* High ⇨ Low
1	Zaire	Argentina	Hungary	Cambodia
2	Nigeria	Croatia	Russian Federation	Bermuda
3	Myanmar	Czech Republic	Mongolia	Azerbaijan
4	Gabon	Costa Rica	Cameroon	India
5	Cambodia	Uruguay	Macedonia, FYR	Mauritania
6	Indonesia	Macedonia, FYR	Croatia	Viet Nam
7	Georgia	Belize	Belarus	Pakistan
8	Pakistan	Jordan	Poland	Paraguay
9	Lao PDR	South Africa	Equatorial Guinea	Uruguay
10	Burundi	Armenia	Czech Republic	El Salvador
11	Guinea	Nicaragua	Bulgaria	Nepal
12	Comoros	Namibia	Comoros	Nigeria
13	Guatemala	Azerbaijan	Sri Lanka	Thailand
14	Cameroon	Panama	Belize	
15	Paraguay	Colombia	Costa Rica	
16	Ethiopia	Brazil	Panama	
17	Guinea-Bissau	Hungary	Algeria	
18	Madagascar	Cambodia	Tonga	
19	Mauritania	Equatorial Guinea		
20	Viet Nam	Venezuela		

Table A.2 Regional Ranking of At-Risk Countries by HNP Indicators

(Maximum ten countries per region)

	Poverty and HNP Outcome Indicators			
Region	*Low GNP per capita*	*High child mortality*	*High child malnutrition*	*High fertility*
East Asia	Cambodia	Cambodia	Vietnam	Lao PDR
	Mongolia	Lao PDR	Indonesia	Solomon Isl.
	Lao PDR	Myanmar	Lao PDR	Vanuatu
	Solomon Isl.	Papua New Guinea	Cambodia	Papua New Guinea
	Kiribati	Indonesia	Myanmar	Cambodia
	Indonesia	Kiribati	Papua New Guinea	Micronesia, FS
	Philippines	Mongolia	Philippines	W. Samoa
	W. Samoa	Philippines	Malaysia	Kiribati
	Papua New Guinea	Solomon Isl.	Solomon Isl.	Philippines
	Vanuatu	Vanuatu		Myanmar
Europe and Central Asia	Tajikistan	Turkmenistan	Turkey	Tajikistan
	Georgia	Turkey	Azerbaijan	Turkmenistan
	Azerbaijan	Tajikistan	Romania	Uzbekistan
	Albania	Uzbekistan		Kyrgyz Rep.
	Kyrgyz Rep.	Kyrgyz Rep.		Turkey
	Armenia	Albania		
	Macedonia, FYR	Kazakhstan		
	Turkmenistan	Macedonia, FYR		
	Uzbekistan	Azerbaijan		
	Bulgaria	Romania		
Latin America & Caribbean	Haiti	Haiti	Guatemala	Guatemala
	Nicaragua	Bolivia	Haiti	Honduras
	Guyana	Guyana	Guyana	Bolivia
	Honduras	Peru	Mexico	Haiti
	Bolivia	Nicaragua	Honduras	Nicaragua
	Suriname	Honduras	Ecuador	Paraguay
	Guatemala	Guatemala	Bolivia	Belize
	Ecuador	Brazil	Nicaragua	El Salvador
	Dominican Rep.	Paraguay	El Salvador	Ecuador
	Jamaica	Belize	Peru	Peru
Middle East & North Africa	Yemen	Iraq	Yemen	Yemen
	Egypt	Yemen	Iran	Gaza
	Morocco	Egypt	Oman	Oman
	Syria	Libya	Iraq	Saudi Arabia
	Jordan	Morocco	Algeria	Libya
	Algeria	Iran	Jordan	Iraq
	Tunisia	Tunisia	Morocco	Syria
	Lebanon	Algeria	Egypt	Jordan
	Oman	Syria	Lebanon	Iran
		Lebanon	Tunisia	Qatar
South Asia	Nepal	Afghanistan	Bangladesh	Afghanistan
	Bangladesh	Bhutan	India	Maldives
	India	Nepal	Nepal	Nepal
	Bhutan	Pakistan	Afghanistan	Pakistan
	Pakistan	Bangladesh	Pakistan	Bangladesh
	Sri Lanka	India	Maldives	India
	Maldives	Maldives	Bhutan	
		Sri Lanka	Sri Lanka	
Sub-Saharan Africa	Mozambique	Liberia	Ethiopia	Niger
	Ethiopia	Sierra Leone	Mauritania	Ethiopia
	Tanzania	Guinea-Bissau	Mozambique	Somalia
	Zaire	Malawi	Niger	Angola
	Burundi	Guinea	Eritrea	Mali
	Malawi	Somalia	Somalia	Burkina Faso
	Chad	Gambia	Burundi	Uganda
	Rwanda	Angola	Angola	Malawi
	Sierra Leone	Rwanda	Nigeria	Liberia
	Niger	Chad	Sudan	Burundi

Region	Coverage Indicators		Health Expenditures Indicators	
	Low immunization	*Low access to health services*	*Low public expenditure/GDP*	*High total health expenditure/GDP*
East Asia	Papua New Guinea	Indonesia	Myanmar	
	Lao PDR	Thailand	Cambodia	
	Myanmar	Malaysia	Indonesia	
	Cambodia		Lao PDR	
	Philippines		Viet Nam	
	Mongolia		Philippines	
			Malaysia	
			Thailand	
			China	
			Korea, Rep.	
Europe and Central Asia	Georgia		Georgia	Croatia
	Latvia		Azerbaijan	Czech Rep.
	Uzbekistan		Kazakhstan	Macedonia, FYR
	Bosnia & Herzegovina		Albania	Armenia
	Russian Fed.		Turkmenistan	Azerbaijan
	Yugoslavia, Fed. Rep.			Hungary
	Kazakhstan			Bulgaria
	Armenia			Belarus
	Kyrgyz Rep.			Poland
	Armenia			
Latin America & Caribbean	Haiti	Haiti	Guatemala	Argentina
	Venezuela	Guatemala	Paraguay	Costa Rica
	Argentina	Honduras	El Salvador	Uruguay
	Brazil	Ecuador	Haiti	Belize
	Paraguay	Panama	Dominican Rep.	Nicaragua
	Guatemala	Colombia	Ecuador	Panama
	Ecuador		Uruguay	Brazil
	Trinidad & Tobago		Venezuela	Colombia
	Costa Rica		Chile	Venezuela
	Nicaragua		Peru	Chile
Middle East & North Africa	Yemen	Morocco	Yemen	Jordan
	Algeria	Iran	Morocco	West Bank/Gaza
	Egypt	Oman	Lebanon	
			Egypt	
			Oman	
			Turkey	
			Iran	
			Tunisia	
South Asia	Pakistan	Bangladesh	Pakistan	
	Nepal	Pakistan	Bangladesh	
			Nepal	
			India	
			Sri Lanka	
			Bhutan	
Sub-Saharan Africa	Chad	Central African Rep.	Nigeria	South Africa
	Niger	Cameroon	Zaire	Namibia
	Angola	Angola	Gabon	Equatorial Guinea
	Zaire	Ghana	Burundi	
	Central African Rep.	Chad	Comoros	
	Cote d'Ivoire	Mozambique	Guinea	
	Sierra Leone	Niger	Cameroon	
	Nigeria	Senegal	Eritrea	
	Eritrea	Benin	Ethiopia	
	Mali	Guinea	Guinea-Bissau	

Table A.3 HNP At A Glance: World Averages

Indicators	World	Low- and middle-income	High income	East Asia & Pacific	Europe & Central Asia	Latin America & Caribbean	Middle East & North Africa	South Asia	Sub-Saharan Africa
Key economic indicators (1995)									
GNP per capita (US$)	4,800	2,650	24,370	830	2,240	3,300	1,780	350	490
GDP (billions US$)	28,403	5,306	21,982	1,418	1,093	1,584	486	435	289
Gross domestic investments/GDP	22	27	21	37	24	20	22	23	20
Present value of debt/GDP	..	29	..	28	25	30	29	27	56
Average annual growth (1990–95)									
GDP	2.0	2.1	2.0	10.3	-6.5	3.2	2.3	4.6	1.4
GNP per capita	0.4	0.3	1.2	8.9	..	1.4	-0.2	2.6	-1.2
Human development (mr 1985–95)									
Secondary school enrollment	..	..	97	55	86	51	59	..	24
Child malnutrition	32	32	..	23	3	11	16	52	30
Urbanization	45	39	78	31	65	74	57	26	31
Access to safe water	71	56	94	67	..	75	79	63	51
Population growth rate	1.4	1.6	0.4	1.2	0.3	1.6	2.5	1.8	2.7
Population under 15, % of total	31	33	19	28	25	35	41	37	45
Health (1995)									
Life expectancy at birth	67	65	77	68	68	69	66	61	51
Percent change, 1980–95	8	13	5	6	1	6	13	15	8
Infant mortality rate	55	60	7	40	26	37	54	75	92
Under-five mortality rate	81	88	9	53	35	47	72	106	157
Adult mortality rate	193	214	97	179	203	148	194	235	397
Nutrition									
Low birth weight (mr 1990–96)	18	19	6	11	..	10	11	33	16
Anemia (mr 1970–95)	..	..	..	..	..	..	..	..	..
Obesity (mr 1976–97)	..	..	..	..	..	..	..	..	..
Reproductive health (mr 1985–95)									
Adolescent fertility rate	60	64	26	25	38	57	68	93	150
Total fertility rate	2.3	3.1	1.7	2.2	2.0	2.8	4.2	3.5	5.7
Percent change, 1980–95	-22	-24	-11	-29	-20	-32	-31	-34	-15
Unwanted fertility rate	..	..	..	..	..	..	..	..	..
Maternal mortality ratio	295	350	14	190	60	170	280	480	870
Future challenges (mr)									
Smear+ Tuberculosis incidence (per 100,000)	58	66	9	56	33	40	30	108	100
Adult HIV/AIDS prevalence (%)	0.6	0.6	0.3	0.1	0.0	0.5	0.0	0.3	4.3
Smoking prevalence (%)	29	29	30	33	41	31	26	23	21
Health services (mr 1990–95)									
In-patient beds per 1,000 population	3.3	2.4	7.6	2.2	9.2	2.3	1.7	0.7	1.2
Physicians per 1,000 population	1.6	1.4	2.4	1.2	3.1	1.4	1.0	0.3	0.1
Access to health services	..	80	..	87	..	79	87	77	53
Immunization coverage, measles	77	76	83	88	80	85	86	73	53
Health finance (mr 1990–95)									
Total health expenditure/GDP	9.1	5.6	9.9	3.5	5.5	7.2	4.4	4.1	5.6
Public health expenditure/GDP	5.5	2.8	6.1	1.5	4.5	3.0	2.7	0.8	2.8
Total health expenditure/cap (US $)	467	62	2329	21	120	234	176	16	42
Total health expenditure/cap (PPP)	525	151	2243	111	272	412	199	72	94

Note: mr (most recent) indicates that data is for the most recent year available or the most recent year within the time period indicated.
.. indicates data not available.

Table A.4 HNP At A Glance: At-Risk Countries, by Region

EAST ASIA AND PACIFIC

	General Indicators			*Poverty and HNP Outcomes*				*Coverage*		*Health Expenditures*	
Indicators	*Low- and middle-income average*	*Regional average (EAP)*	*Largest population (China)*	*Low GNP per capita (Cambodia)*	*High under-5 mortality (Laos)*	*High child malnutrition (Vietnam)*	*High fertility rate (Solomon Islands)*	*Low immunization (Papua New Guinea)*	*Low access to health services (Indonesia)*	*Low public expenditure % of GDP (Myanmar)*	*High total expenditure % of GDP (*)*
Key economic indicators (1995)											
GNP per capita (US$)	2,650	830	620	270	350	..	910	1,160	980	..	
Gross domestic investments/GDP	27	37	41	15	..	24	..	19	35	13	
Present value of debt/GDP	29	28	16	69	43	137	..	46	51	..	
Average annual growth (1990–95)											
GDP	2.1	10.3	12.9	6.4	6.5	8.3	..	9.3	7.6	5.7	
GNP per capita (1985–95)	0.3	8.9	11.4	..	3.2	..	2.2	6.0	6.0	..	
Human development (mr 1985–95)											
Secondary school enrollment	..	55	52		25	35	..	12	43	..	
Child malnutrition	32	23	16	38	40	45	21	30	40	31	
Urbanization	39	31	30	21	22	21	17	16	34	26	
Access to safe water	56	67	46	13	41	38	..	31	63	39	
Gini index	..	..	38	..	30	36	..	..	32	..	
Population growth rate	1.6	1.2	1.1	2.8	3.0	2.0	3.0	2.3	1.6	1.7	
Population under 15, % of total	33	28	26	44	45	37	43	39	33	36	
Health (1995)											
Life expectancy at birth	65	68	69	53	53	67	63	57	64	59	
Percent change, 1980–95	13	6	4	35	16	8	..	12	18	13	
Infant mortality rate	60	40	35	109	92	41	41	65	52	84	
Under-five mortality rate	88	53	43	158	147	49	52	95	75	119	
Adult mortality rate	214	179	164	334	410	171	284	355	235	280	
Nutrition											
Low birth weight (mr 1990–96)	19	11	6	..	18	17	..	23	14	16	
Anemia (mr 1970–95)	..	..	52	..	..	52	..	13	64	58	
Obesity (mr 1976–97)	..	..	4.3	..	0.7	..	..	1.6	..	..	
Reproductive health (mr 1985–95)											
Adolescent fertility rate	64	25	17	108	59	42	94	44	57	30	
Total fertility rate	3.1	2.2	1.9	4.7	6.7	5.1	6.8	5.7	2.7	3.5	
Percent change, 1980–95	-24	-29	-24	3	-2	-39	-23	-15	-38	-26	
Unwanted fertility rate	..	..	..	..	..	..	..	..	0.5	..	
Maternal mortality ratio	350	190	115	900	660	105	..	930	390	518	
Future challenges (mr)											
Smear+ Tuberculosis incid. (per 100,000)	66	56	38	106	105	75	54	124	99	85	
Adult HIV/AIDS prevalence (%)	0.6	0.1	0.0	1.9	0.0	0.1	..	0.2	0.1	1.5	
Smoking prevalence (%)	29	33	34	..	28	39	..	37	29	..	
Health services (mr 1990–95)											
In-patient beds per 1,000 pop.	2.4	2.2	2.4	2.1	2.5	3.8	2.8	4.0	0.7	0.6	
Physicians per 1,000 pop.	1.4	1.2	1.6	0.1	0.2	0.4	0.2	0.1	0.2	0.1	
Access to health services, %	80	..	..	..	..	97	..	96	43	..	
Immunization coverage, measles,%	76	88	89	75	65	93	..	35	89	66	
Health finance (mr 1990–95)											
Total health expenditure/GDP	5.6	3.5	3.8	7.2	2.6	5.2	5.6	..	1.5	..	
Public health expenditure/GDP	2.8	1.5	1.8	0.7	0.8	1.1	3.3	2.8	0.7	0.4	
Total health expenditure/cap (US$)	62	21	19	18	10	..	39	..	14	..	
Total health expenditure/cap (PPP)	151	111	98	..	..	..	111	..	63	..	

Note: * indicates no country within the Region fits the profile.

Table A.4 (*continued*)

EUROPE AND CENTRAL ASIA											
	General Indicators			*Poverty and HNP Outcomes*				*Coverage*		*Health Expenditures*	
Indicators	*Low- and middle-income average*	*Regional average (ECA)*	*Largest population (Russia)*	*Low GNP per capita (Tajikistan)*	*High under-5 mortality (Turkmen-istan)*	*High child malnutrition (Turkey)*	*High fertility rate (Uzbek-istan)*	*Low immu-nization (Georgia)*	*Low access to health services (*)*	*Low public expenditure % of GDP (Azerbaijan)*	*High total expenditure % of GDP (Croatia)*
Key economic indicators (1995)											
GNP per capita (US$)	2,650	2,240	2,240	340	920	2,780	970	440		480	3,250
Gross domestic investments/GDP	27	24	28	21	..	24	31	3		16	14
Present value of debt/GDP	29	25	26	22	8	40	6	37		4	17
Average annual growth (1990–95)											
GDP	2.1	-6.5	-9.8	-18.1	-10.6	3.2	-4.4	-26.9		-20.2	..
GNP per capita	0.3	..	-10.2	-20.3	..	1.5	-6.4	-25.1		-21.0	..
Human development (mr 1985–95)											
Secondary school enrollment	..	86	88	100	..	61	94	..		88	83
Child malnutrition	32	3	..	..	..	10	4	..		1-	..
Urbanization	39	65	73	32	45	69	41	58		56	64
Access to safe water	56	..	..	..	85	92	..	..		..	82
Gini index	..	..	..	..	..	..	..	..		..	..
Population growth rate	1.6	0.3	-0.1	1.6	4.5	1.6	2.1	-0.3		0.9	-0.0
Population under 15, % of total	33	25	21	43	39	33	41	23		33	19
Health (1995)											
Life expectancy at birth	65	68	65	66	..	68	..	73		70	74
Percent change, 1980–95	13	1	-2	-3	..	11	..	4		3	5
Infant mortality rate	60	26	18	42	46	49	30	18		25	16
Under-five mortality rate	88	35	21	61	65	63	48	21		31	18
Adult mortality rate	214	203	286	199	186	135	155	133		161	127
Nutrition											
Low birth weight (mr 1990–96)	19	..	..	..	..	8	..	..		..	8
Anemia (mr 1970–95)	..	..	30	50	..	..	..	..		..	..
Obesity (mr 1976–97)	..	..	..	..	..	..	7.8	..		..	..
Reproductive health (mr 1985–95)											
Adolescent fertility rate	64	38	31	48	26	44	43	40		33	28
Total fertility rate	3.1	2.0	1.4	4.2	3.8	2.7	3.7	..		2.3	1.5
Percent change, 1980–95	-24	-20	-26	-26	-24	-37	-23	..		-28	..
Unwanted fertility rate	..	..	..	..	..	..	..	..		..	..
Maternal mortality ratio	350	60	52	39	43	183	43	55		29	10
Future challenges (mr)											
Smear+ Tuberculosis incid. (per 100,000)	66	33	45	60	32	26	25	32		21	29
Adult HIV/AIDS prevalence (%)	0.6	0.0	0.0	0.0	0.0	0.0	0.0	0.0		0.0	0.0
Smoking prevalence (%)	29	41	49	..	14	44	21	43		..	38
Health services (mr 1990–95)											
In-patient beds per 1,000 pop.	2.4	9.2	11.7	8.8	10.5	2.5	8.4	8.2		10.0	5.9
Physicians per 1,000 pop	1.4	3.1	3.8	2.1	3.2	1.1	3.3	4.1		3.9	2.0
Access to health services, %	80	..	..	..	..	100	..	..			..
Immunization coverage, measles,%	76	80	91	90	90	75	71	63			90
Health finance (mr 1990–95)											
Total health expenditure/GDP	5.6	5.5	4.8	..	..	4.2	..	..		7.5	10.1
Public health expenditure/GDP	2.8	4.5	4.1	6.4	2.8	2.7	3.5	0.8		1.4	8.5
Total health expenditure/cap (US$)	62	120	96	..	..	99	..	..		32	302
Total health expenditure/cap (PPP)	151	272	225	..	..	239	..	..		96	..

LATIN AMERICA AND THE CARIBBEAN											
	General Indicators			*Poverty and HNP Outcomes*				*Coverage*		*Health Expenditures*	
Indicators	*Low- and middle-income average*	*Regional average (LAC)*	*Largest population (Brazil)*	*Low GNP per capita (Haiti)*	*High under-5 mortality (Bolivia)*	*High child malnutrition (Guatemala)*	*High fertility rate (Honduras)*	*Low immunization (Haiti)*	*Low access to health services (Guatemala)*	*Low public expenditure % of GDP (Guatemala)*	*High total expenditure % of GDP (Argentina)*
Key economic indicators (1995)											
GNP per capita (US$)	2,650	3,300	3,640	250	800	1,340	600	250	1,340	1,340	8,030
Gross domestic investments/GDP	27	20	21	3	15	18	26	3	18	18	19
Present value of debt/GDP	29	30	27	24	62	20	96	24	20	20	27
Average annual growth (1990–95)											
GDP	2.1	3.2	2.7	-6.5	3.8	4.0	3.5	-6.5	4.0	4.0	5.7
GNP per capita	0.3	1.4	1.0	-8.4	1.8	0.0	1.1	-8.4	0.0	0.0	4.9
Human development (mr 1985–95)											
Secondary school enrollment	..	51	43	..	..	24	32	..	24	24	72
Child malnutrition	32	11	7	28	16	33	18	28	33	33	2
Urbanization	39	74	78	32	58	42	48	32	42	42	88
Access to safe water	56	75	92	28	60	64	70	28	64	64	64
Gini index	..	..	63	..	42	60	53	..	60	60	..
Population growth rate	1.6	1.6	1.4	2.1	2.4	2.9	3.0	2.1	2.9	2.9	1.3
Population under 15, % of total	33	35	32	40	41	44	44	40	44	44	29
Health (1995)											
Life expectancy at birth	65	69	67	56	60	65	67	56	65	65	73
Percent change, 1980–95	13	6	8	8	15	14	11	8	14	14	5
Infant mortality rate	60	37	45	73	70	45	46	73	45	45	22
Under-five mortality rate	88	47	57	101	96	58	59	101	58	58	27
Adult mortality rate	214	148	152	360	264	206	138	360	206	206	130
Nutrition											
Low birth weight (mr 1990–96)	19	10	11	15	12	14	..	15	14	14	6
Anemia (mr 1970–95)	..	..	33	..	54	..	14	..	..	..	26
Obesity (mr 1976–97)	..	..	5.4	..	..	2.8	1.8	..	2.8	2.8	7.0
Reproductive health (mr 1985–95)											
Adolescent fertility rate	64	57	37	70	82	106	112	70	106	106	62
Total fertility rate	3.1	2.8	2.4	4.5	4.6	4.8	4.7	4.5	4.8	4.8	2.7
Percent change, 1980–95	-24	-32	-38	-24	-17	-23	-28	-24	-23	-23	-17
Unwanted fertility rate	..	..	..	1.8	1.9	..	..	1.8	..	..	..
Maternal mortality ratio	350	170	200	600	373	464	220	600	464	464	100
Future challenges (mr)											
Smear+ Tuberculosis incid. (per 100,000)	66	40	36	150	151	49	60	150	49	49	22
Adult HIV/AIDS prevalence (%)	0.6	0.5	0.7	4.4	0.1	0.4	1.6	4.4	0.4	0.4	0.4
Smoking prevalence (%)	29	31	33	..	36	31	24	..	31	31	32
Health services (mr 1990–95)											
In-patient beds per 1,000 pop.	2.4	2.3	3.0	0.8	1.4	1.1	1.0	0.8	1.1	1.1	4.6
Physicians per 1,000 pop.	1.4	1.4	..	0.1	0.5	0.8	0.4	0.1	0.8	0.8	2.7
Access to health services, %	80	79	..	45	..	60	62	45	60	60	..
Immunization coverage, measles,%	76	85	78	24	83	84	90	24	84	84	76
Health finance (mr 1990–95)											
Total health expenditure/GDP	5.6	7.2	7.4	3.6	5.0	2.7	5.6	3.6	2.7	2.7	10.6
Public health expenditure/GDP	2.8	3.0	2.7	1.3	2.7	0.9	2.8	1.3	0.9	0.9	4.3
Total health expenditure/cap (US$)	62	234	261	8	38	33	34	8	33	33	877
Total health expenditure/cap (PPP)	151	412	428	35	138	92	121	35	92	92	932

Table A.4 (*continued*)

MIDDLE EAST AND NORTH AFRICA											
	General Indicators			*Poverty and HNP Outcomes*				*Coverage*		*Health Expenditures*	
Indicators	*Low- and middle-income average*	*Regional average (MENA)*	*Largest population (Iran)*	*Low GNP per capita (Yemen)*	*High under-5 mortality (Iraq)*	*High child malnutrition (Oman)*	*High fertility rate (Gaza)*	*Low immu-nization (Yemen)*	*Low access to health services (Morocco)*	*Low public expenditure % of GDP (Yemen)*	*High total expenditure % of GDP (Jordan)*
Key economic indicators (1995)											
GNP per capita (US$)	2,650	1,780	..	260	..	4,820	..	260	1,110	260	1,510
Gross domestic investments/GDP	27	22	28	14	..	..	..	14	15	14	31
Present value of debt/GDP	29	29	..	108	..	24	..	108	65	108	103
Average annual growth (1990–95)											
GDP	2.1	2.3	4.2	..	..	6.0	..	..	1.2	..	8.2
GNP per capita	0.3	-0.2	1.2	..	..	-0.8	..	..	-0.8	..	3.6
Human development (mr 1985–95)											
Secondary school enrollment	..	59	66	44	61	..	..	44	24	44	53
Child malnutrition	32	16	17	30	12	14	..	30	10	30	10
Urbanization	39	57	59	34	75	13	95	34	48	34	71
Access to safe water	56	79	89	52	45	56	..	52	59	52	89
Gini index	..	..	..	..	..	..	..	..	39	..	43
Population growth rate	1.6	2.5	2.7	3.2	2.1	5.5	6.3	3.2	2.0	3.2	4.3
Population under 15, % of total	33	41	44	48	44	46	48	48	36	48	42
Health (1995)											
Life expectancy at birth	65	66	68	53	61	70	..	53	66	53	70
Percent change, 1980–95	13	13	13	9	-1	20	..	9	14	9	..
Infant mortality rate	60	54	46	101	111	18	31	101	56	101	31
Under-five mortality rate	88	72	59	145	145	22	51	145	75	145	33
Adult mortality rate	214	194	154	358	162	167	125	358	188	358	145
Nutrition											
Low birth weight (mr 1990–96)	19	11	12	19	15	10	..	19	9	19	7
Anemia (mr 1970–95)	..	..	..	..	18	54	..	..	45	..	..
Obesity (mr 1976–97)	..	..	..	..	..	..	..	..	5	..	..
Reproductive health (mr 1985–95)											
Adolescent fertility rate	64	68	80	141	61	123	119	141	38	141	43
Total fertility rate	3.1	4.2	4.6	7.4	5.5	7.1	7.1	7.4	3.5	7.4	4.8
Percent change, 1980–95	-24	-31	-26	-6	-15	-29	3	-6	-36	-6	-30
Unwanted fertility rate	..	..	..	1.7	..	..	..	1.7	1.4	1.7	1.6
Maternal mortality ratio	350	280	120	1470	310	190	..	1470	372	1470	132
Future challenges (mr)											
Smear+ Tuberculosis incid. (per 100,000)	66	30	23	43	67	9	..	43	56	43	6
Adult HIV/AIDS prevalence (%)	0.6	0.0	0.0	0.0	0.0	0.1	..	0.0	0.0	0.0	0.0
Smoking prevalence (%)	29	26	..	..	..	..	..	..	24	..	45
Health services (mr 1990–95)											
In -patient beds per 1,000 pop.	2.4	1.7	1.4	0.8	1.7	..	..	0.8	1.1	0.8	1.6
Physicians per 1,000 pop.	1.4	1.0	..	0.1	0.2	..	..	0.1	0.4	0.1	1.6
Access to health services, %	80	87	73	..	98	89	..	..	62	..	90
Immunization coverage, measles,%	76	86	95	49	95	98	..	49	92	49	92
Health finance (mr 1990–95)											
Total health expenditure/GDP	5.6	4.4	4.8	2.6	..	..	..	2.6	3.4	2.6	7.9
Public health expenditure/GDP	2.8	2.7	2.8	1.1	..	2.5	..	1.1	1.6	1.1	3.7
Total health expenditure/cap (US$)	62	176	467	39	-	..	..	39	36	39	118
Total health expenditure/cap (PPP)	151	199	239	..	..	..	..	..	126	..	347

SOUTH ASIA

Indicators	General Indicators			Poverty and HNP Outcomes				Coverage		Health Expenditures	
	Low- and middle-income average	*Regional average (SAS)*	*Largest population (India)*	*Low GNP per capita (Nepal)*	*High under-5 mortality (Afghanistan)*	*High child malnutrition (Bangladesh)*	*High fertility rate (Maldives)*	*Low immunization (Pakistan)*	*Low access to health services (Bangladesh)*	*Low public expenditure % of GDP (Pakistan)*	*High total expenditure % of GDP (*)*
Key economic indicators (1995)											
GNP per capita (US$)	2,650	350	340	200	..	240	990	460	240	460	
Gross domestic investments/GDP	27	23	23	23	..	15	..	20	15	20	
Present value of debt/GDP	29	27	25	28	..	33	..	40	33	40	
Average annual growth (1990–95)											
GDP	2.1	4.6	4.6	5.1	..	4.1	..	4.6	4.1	4.6	
GNP per capita	0.3	2.6	2.8	2.6	..	2.6	3.9	1.0	2.6	1.0	
Human development (mr 1985–95)											
Secondary school enrollment	..	..	..	21	..	19	..	..	19	..	
Child malnutrition	32	52	53	49	40	68	39	40	68	40	
Urbanization	39	26	27	14	20	18	33	35	18	35	
Access to safe water	56	63	63	48	..	83	..	60	83	60	
Gini index	..	..	34	30	..	28	..	31	28	31	
Population growth rate	1.6	1.8	1.7	2.5	2.8	1.6	3.2	2.9	1.6	2.9	
Population under 15, % of total	33	37	35	42	44	43	45	43	43	43	
Health (1995)											
Life expectancy at birth	65	61	62	56	45	58	63	63	58	63	
Percent change, 1980–95	13	15	17	19	11	22	15	15	22	15	
Infant mortality rate	60	75	69	92	159	80	53	91	80	91	
Under-five mortality rate	88	106	95	131	237	115	70	127	115	127	
Adult mortality rate	214	235	224	340	420	303	235	218	303	218	
Nutrition											
Low birth weight (mr 1990–96)	19	33	33	26	20	34	..	25	34	25	
Anemia (mr 1970–95)	..	..	88	65	..	53	20	37	53	37	
Obesity (mr 1976–97)	..	..	0.5	..	..	0.3	..	..	0.3	..	
Reproductive health (mr 1985–95)											
Adolescent fertility rate	64	93	81	82	153	116	76	107	116	107	
Total fertility rate	3.1	3.5	3.2	5.3	6.9	3.5	6.7	5.3	3.5	5.3	
Percent change, 1980–95	-24	-34	-35	-17	-2	-43	-4	-24	-43	-24	
Unwanted fertility rate	..	..	0.8	..	..	1.3	..	1.2	1.3	1.2	
Maternal mortality ratio	350	480	437	515	1,700	887	..	340	887	340	
Future challenges (mr)											
Smear+ Tuberculosis incid. (per 100,000)	66	108	99	75	125	99	54	67	99	67	
Adult HIV/AIDS prevalence	0.6	0.3	0.4	0.1	0.0	0.0	0.1	0.1	0.0	0.1	
Smoking prevalence	29	23	22	..	..	38	..	16	38	16	
Health services (mr 1990–95)											
In-patient beds per 1,000 pop.	2.4	0.7	0.8	0.2	0.2	0.3	0.8	0.7	0.3	0.7	
Physicians per 1,000 pop.	1.4	0.3	..	0.1	0.1	0.2	0.1	0.5	0.2	0.5	
Access to health services, %	80	77	..	..	..	74	..	85	74	85	
Immunization coverage, measles,%	76	73	84	78	19	96	86	53	96	53	
Health finance (mr 1990–95)											
Total health expenditure/GDP	5.6	4.1	5.6	5.0	..	2.4	4.9	3.5	2.4	3.5	
Public health expenditure/GDP	2.8	0.8	1.2	1.2	..	1.2	..	0.8	1.2	0.8	
Total health expenditure/cap (US$)	62	16	11	10	..	6	..	13	6	13	
Total health expenditure/cap (PPP)	151	72	44	60	..	35	..	70	35	70	

Table A.4 (*continued*)

SUB-SAHARAN AFRICA											
	General Indicators			*Poverty and HNP Outcomes*				*Coverage*		*Health Expenditures*	
Indicators	*Low- and middle-income average*	*Regional average (SSA)*	*Largest population (Nigeria)*	*Low GNP per capita (Mozambique)*	*High under-5 mortality (Liberia)*	*High child malnutrition (Ethiopia)*	*High fertility rate (Niger)*	*Low immunization (Chad)*	*Low access to health services (CAR)*	*Low public expenditure % of GDP (Nigeria)*	*High total expenditure % of GDP (S. Africa)*
Key economic indicators (1995)											
GNP per capita (US$)	2,650	490	260	80	..	100	220	180	340	260	3,160
Gross domestic investments/GDP	27	20	20	58	..	16	..	..	13	20	17
Present value of debt/GDP	29	56	106	281	..	60	52	38	45	106	..
Average annual growth (1990–95)											
GDP	2.1	1.4	1.6	7.1	..	..	0.5	1.9	1.0	1.6	0.6
GNP per capita	0.3	-1.2	1.1	4.1	..	1.0	-2.6	-0.1	-2.2	1.1	-1.1
Human development (mr 1985–95)											
Secondary school enrollment	..	24	..	..	..	..	..	..	..	..	..
Child malnutrition	32	30	35	47	20	48	43	..	23	35	9
Urbanization	39	31	39	34	45	13	23	21	39	39	51
Access to safe water	56	51	43	28	..	27	57	29	..	43	..
Gini index	..	..	38	..	..	..	36	..	..	38	59
Population growth rate	1.6	2.7	2.9	2.9	2.4	2.7	3.3	2.5	2.2	2.9	2.2
Population under 15, % of total	33	45	45	44	45	47	48	43	43	45	37
Health (1995)											
Life expectancy at birth	65	51	53	47	46	49	47	49	49	53	64
Percent change, 1980–95	13	8	15	4	-12	16	14	14	6	15	12
Infant mortality rate	60	92	81	114	177	113	120	118	98	81	51
Under-five mortality rate	88	157	176	190	239	188	..	197	160	176	67
Adult mortality rate	214	397	414	385	225	397	456	428	456	414	..
Nutrition											
Low birth weight (mr 1990–96)	19	16	16	20	..	16	15	..	15	16	..
Anemia (mr 1970–95)	..	..	55	58	78	42	41	37	67	55	37
Obesity (mr 1976–97)	..	..	..	..	..	..	..	..	4.8	..	..
Reproductive health (mr 1985–95)											
Adolescent fertility rate	64	150	120	122	211	164	222	183	145	120	68
Total fertility rate	3.1	5.7	5.5	6.2	6.6	7.0	7.4	5.9	5.1	5.5	3.9
Percent change, 1980–95	-24	-15	-18	-3	-3	8	0	0	-12	-18	-20
Unwanted fertility rate	..	..	1.0	..	0.6	..	0.3	..	0.4	1.0	..
Maternal mortality ratio	350	870	1,000	1,510	560	1,530	593	1,590	650	1,000	404
Future challenges (mr)											
Smear+ Tuberculosis incid. (per 100,000)	66	100	100	85	45	70	65	75	63	100	112
Adult HIV/AIDS prevalence (%)	0.6	4.3	2.2	5.8	1.3	2.5	1.0	2.7	5.8	2.2	3.2
Smoking prevalence (%)	29	..	16	..	..	..	..	..	..	16	35
Health services (mr 1990–95)											
In-patient beds per 1,000 pop.	2.4	1.2	1.7	0.9	..	0.2	..	0.7	0.9	1.7	..
Physicians per 1,000 pop.	1.4	0.1	..	..	..	..	0.0	..	0.0	..	..
Access to health services, %	80	53	67	30	..	55	30	26	13	67	..
Immunization coverage, measles,%	76	53	50	71	..	54	38	24	70	50	76
Health finance (mr 1990–95)											
Total health expenditure/GDP	5.6	5.6	1.4	..	..	..	..	..	..	1.4	7.9
Public health expenditure/GDP	2.8	2.5	0.3	4.6	..	1.1	1.6	2.5	1.9	0.3	3.6
Total health expenditure/cap (US$)	62	42	5	..	..	..	..	9	..	5	233
Total health expenditure/cap (PPP)	151	94	18	..	..	..	..	29	..	18	396

Note: .. indicates data not available.

Table A.5 HNP At A Glance: At-Risk Countries Amoung High-Income Countries

	HIGH-INCOME COUNTRIES										
	General Indicators			*Poverty and HNP Outcomes*				*Coverage*		*Health Expenditures*	
Indicators	*Low- and middle-income average*	*Regional average (high-income)*	*Largest population (USA)*	*Low GNP per capita (Portugal)*	*High under-5 mortality (Qatar)*	*High child malnutrition (*)*	*High fertility rate (UAE)*	*Low immu-nization (Italy)*	*Low access to health services (*)*	*Low public expenditure % of GDP (Singapore)*	*High total expenditure % of GDP (USA)*
Key economic indicators (1995)											
GNP per capita (US$)	2,650	24,370	26,980	9,740	11,600		17,400	19,020		26,730	26,980
Gross domestic investments/GDP	27	21	..	..	..		25.3	17.4		34.9	..
Present value of debt/GDP	29	..	..	..	..		..	..		..	..
Average annual growth (1990–95)											
GDP	2.1	2.0	2.6	0.8	..		..	1.0		8.7	2.6
GNP per capita	0.3	1.2	1.5	0.7	-5.1		-4.8	0.7		6.4	1.5
Human development (1985–95)											
Secondary school enrollment	..	97	97	81	..		89	81		78	97
Child malnutrition	32	..	..	..	6		7	..		..	..
Urbanization	39	78	76	36	91		84	67		100	75
Access to safe water	56	94	90	..	..		95	..		100	90
Gini index	..	..	..	..	..		..	..		..	..
Population growth rate	1.6	0.4	1.0	0.1	5.8		5.0	0.2		1.9	1.0
Population under 15, % of total	33	19	22	19	30		29	15		24	22
Health (1995)											
Life expectancy at birth	65	77	77	75	72		75	78		77	77
Percent change, 1980–95	13	5	4	6	8		10	5		7	4
Infant mortality rate	60	7	8	7	19		16	7		4	8
Under-five mortality rate	88	9	10	11	22		19	8		6	10
Adult mortality rate	214	97	123	120	140		110	91		103	123
Nutrition											
Low birth weight (mr 1990–96)	19	6	7	5	..		..	..		7	7
Anemia (mr 1970–95)	..	..	..	..	..		46	..		..	..
Obesity (mr 1976–97)	..	..	..	..	..		..	..		..	..
Reproductive health (mr 1985–95)											
Adolescent fertility rate	64	26	60	23	40		58	14		13	60
Total fertility rate	3.1	1.7	2.1	1.4	3.9		3.6	1.2		1.7	2.1
Percent change, 1980–95	-24	-11	+17	-36	-33		-33	-25		0	+17
Unwanted fertility rate	..	..	..	..	..		..	..		..	..
Maternal mortality ratio	350	14	12	15	..		33	12		10	12
Future challenges (mr)											
Smear+ Tuberculosis incid. (per 100,000)	66	9	4	27	23		13	11		37	4
Adult HIV/AIDS prevalence (%)	0.6	0.3	0.5	0.2	..		0.0	0.3		0.1	0.5
Smoking prevalence (%)	29	30	25	27	..		..	38		17	25
Health services (1990–95)											
In-patient beds per 1,000 pop.	2.4	7.6	4.4	4.3	..		3.1	6.7		3.6	4.4
Physicians per 1,000 pop	1.4	2.4	2.5	2.9	1.5		0.8	1.7		1.4	2.5
Access to health services, %	80	..	..	100	..		90	..		100	..
Immunization coverage, measles,%	76	83	89	94	87		90	50		88	89
Health finance (mr 1990–95)											
Total health expenditure/GDP	5.6	9.9	14.5	8.1	2.8		2.2	7.7		3.5	14.5
Public health expenditure/GDP	2.8	6.1	7.0	4.5	..		1.9	5.4		1.1	7.0
Total health expenditure/cap (US$)	62	2,329	3,828	287	343		379	1,471		621	3,828
Total health expenditure/cap (PPP)	151	2,243	3,828	1,058	511		378	1,605		823	3,873

Note: .. indicates data not available.
* indicates no country within the Region fits the profile.

Table A.6 HNP At A Glance: Indicators by Country

Country	Key Economic Indicators		Average Annual Growth		Human Development						
	GNP/cap. 1995 (US$)	Central gov. exp. 1994–95 (US $ millions)	GDP 1990–95 (percent)	GNP/cap. 1990–95 (percent)	Population 1995 (millions)	Population growth rate 1995 (percent)	Gross sec. school enrollment mr 1985–95 (% of age group)	Child malnutrition mr 1985–95 (% of under-5 age group)	Urbanization mr 1985–95 (% of pop.)	Access to safe water mr 1985–95 (percent)	Gini index mr 1985–95 (percent)
Afghanistan	..	..	..	..	23.5	2.8	15	40	20	..	..
Albania	670	752	1.4	..	3.3	0.0	..	..	37	..	..
Algeria	1600	..	0.1	-2.3	28.0	2.2	61	10	56	..	38.7
Angola	410	..	-4.1	-6.6	10.8	3.1	14	35	32	32	..
Anguilla	..	..	..	..	..	..	..	..	..	..	..
Antigua and Barbuda	..	..	..	..	0.1	0.4	..	..	35	..	..
Argentina	8030	..	5.7	4.9	34.7	1.3	..	2	88	64	..
Armenia	730	..	-21.2	-20.7	3.8	1.0	85	..	69	..	..
Aruba	..	..	..	..	0.1	0.9	..	..	..	..	..
Australia	18720	96366	3.5	2.6	18.1	1.1	84	..	85	95	..
Austria	26890	80198	1.9	1.1	8.1	0.7	107	..	56	..	..
Azerbaijan	480	..	-20.2	-21.0	7.5	0.9	88	10	56	..	..
Bahamas, The	11940	..	..	-1.9	0.3	1.6	91	..	87	..	..
Bahrain	7840	1580	..	3.8	0.6	3.2	99	7	90	..	..
Bangladesh	240	..	4.1	2.6	119.8	1.6	19	68	18	83	28.3
Barbados	6560	..	..	-1.0	0.3	0.8	..	6	48	..	..
Belarus	2070	..	-9.3	-9.9	10.3	0.2	92	..	71	..	21.6
Belgium	24710	114776	1.1	1.1	10.1	0.4	..	..	97	..	..
Belize	..	180	..	0.9	0.2	2.6	38	6	47	..	..
Benin	370	..	4.1	1.6	5.5	2.9	..	24	42	70	..
Bermuda	..	..	..	..	0.1	0.8	..	..	..	..	..
Bhutan	420	146	..	1.8	0.7	..	..	38	..	..	..
Bolivia	800	1417	3.8	1.8	7.4	2.4	..	16	58	60	42.0
Bosnia & Herzegovina	..	..	..	..	4.4	0.0	..	..	49	..	..
Botswana	3020	..	4.2	2.6	1.5	2.4	19	27	31	70	..
Brazil	3640	..	2.7	1.0	159.2	1.4	43	7	78	92	63.4
Brunei	25160	..	..	..	0.3	1.9	71	..	59		..
Bulgaria	1330	5374	-4.3	-2.4	8.4	-0.7	72	..	71	..	30.8
Burkina Faso	230	..	2.6	-0.4	10.4	2.8	8	33	27	..	..
Burundi	160	..	-2.3	-4.9	6.3	2.6	7	38	8	58	..
Cambodia	270	..	6.4	..	10.0	2.8	29	38	21	13	..
Cameroon	650	..	-1.8	-4.6	13.3	2.9	..	15	45	41	..
Canada	19380	..	1.8	0.5	29.6	1.3	88	..	77	100	..
Cape Verde	960	..	..	3.9	0.4	2.2	8	19	54	..	..
Cayman Islands	..	..	..	..	..	..	..	..	..	..	..
Central African Republic	340	..	1.0	-2.2	3.3	2.2	..	23	39	..	..
Chad	180	..	1.9	-0.1	6.4	2.5	9	..	21	29	..
Channel Islands	..	..	..	..	0.1	-0.1	..	..	29	..	..
Chile	4160	12954	7.3	6.3	14.2	1.5	70	1	86	96	56.5
China	620	51052	12.8	11.4	1203.3	1.1	52	16	30	46	41.5
Colombia	1910	..	4.6	3.2	36.8	1.8	62	8	73	96	51.3
Comoros	470	..	..	-1.7	0.5	2.9	19	..	28	..	..
Congo	680	..	-0.6	-5.2	2.6	2.9	..	24	59	60	..
Costa Rica	2610	2626	5.1	3.0	3.4	2.4	47	2	50	100	46.1
Cote d'Ivoire	660	..	0.7	-2.5	14.0	3.0	25	24	44	..	36.9
Croatia	3250	8403	..	..	4.8	0.0	83	..	64	82	..
Cuba	..	..	..	..	11.0	0.6	77	8	76	96	..
Cyprus	..	2418	..	..	0.7	1.4	95	..	54	..	..
Czech Republic	3870	18801	-2.6	-2.6	10.3	0.1	86	1	65	94	26.6
Denmark	29890	74968	2.0	1.8	5.2	0.3	114	..	85	100	..
Djibouti	..	..	..	..	0.6	4.9	12	23	83	..	..
Dominica	2990	..	..	2.2	0.1	0.3	..	..	..	..	..
Dominican Republic	1460	1786	3.9	3.0	7.8	1.9	37	10	65	79	50.5
Ecuador	1390	2604	3.4	0.9	11.5	2.2	55	17	58	70	46.6
Egypt, Arab Republic	790	..	1.3	-0.1	57.8	1.9	76	9	45	84	32.0
El Salvador	1610	1180	6.3	4.6	5.6	2.3	29	11	45	62	..
Equatorial Guinea	380	..	..	4.1	0.4	2.8	..	..	42	..	..

Country	Key Economic Indicators: GNP/cap. 1995 (US$)	Key Economic Indicators: Central gov. exp. 1994–95 (US $ millions)	Average Annual Growth: GDP 1990–95 (percent)	Average Annual Growth: GNP/cap. 1990–95 (percent)	Human Development: Population 1995 (millions)	Population growth rate 1995 (percent)	Gross sec. school enrollment mr 1985–95 (% of age group)	Child malnutrition mr 1985–95 (% of under-5 age group)	Urbanization mr 1985–95 (% of pop.)	Access to safe water mr 1985–95 (percent)	Gini index mr 1985–95 (percent)
Eritrea	..	..	..	..	3.6	2.6	14	41	17	..	..
Estonia	2860	738	-9.2	-7.7	1.5	-1.3	92	..	73	..	39.5
Ethiopia	100	1402	..	1.0	56.4	2.7	11	48	13	27	..
Fiji	2440	570	..	1.2	0.8	1.1	64	8	41	..	..
Finland	20580	42692	-0.5	-1.3	5.1	0.5	119	..	63	100	..
France	24990	713215	1.0	0.5	58.1	0.4	106	..	73	100	..
French Guiana	..	..	..	..	..	..	..	..	..	..	..
French Polynesia	..	..	..	..	0.2	2.7	77	..	..	..	..
Gabon	3490	..	-2.5	-7.9	1.1	2.5	..	15	50	67	..
Gambia, The	320	..	1.6	-4.7	1.1	3.6	19	17	26	61	..
Gaza Strip	..	..	..	..	0.9	6.3	..	..	95	..	..
Georgia	440	..	-26.9	-25.1	5.4	-0.3	..	..	58	..	..
Germany	27510	816395	..	..	81.9	0.6	101	..	87	..	..
Ghana	390	..	4.3	1.4	17.1	2.7	..	27	36	56	33.9
Greece	8210	..	1.1	0.8	10.5	0.5	..	..	65	..	..
Grenada	2980	78	..	..	0.1	..	..	..	..	..	..
Guadeloupe	..	..	..	..	0.4	1.5	..	..	51	..	..
Guam	..	..	..	..	0.1	2.3	..	..	38	..	..
Guatemala	1340	1156	4.0	0.0	10.6	2.9	24	33	42	64	59.6
Guinea	550	..	3.8	2.0	6.6	2.7	12	24	30	49	46.8
Guinea-Bissau	250	..	3.5	0.4	1.1	2.1	6	23	22	57	56.2
Guyana	590	..	..	10.9	0.8	1.0	57	27	36	..	..
Haiti	250	..	-6.5	-8.4	7.2	2.1	..	28	32	28	..
Honduras	600	..	3.5	1.1	5.9	3.0	32	18	48	70	52.7
Hong Kong	22990	..	5.6	3.9	6.2	1.8	..	..	95	..	..
Hungary	4120	..	-1.0	-1.3	10.2	-0.3	81	..	65	..	27.0
Iceland	24950	2044	..	-0.2	0.3	1.0	103	..	92	..	..
India	340	53659	4.6	2.8	929.4	1.7	..	53	27	63	33.8
Indonesia	980	28647	7.6	6.0	193.3	1.6	43	40	34	63	31.7
Iran, Islamic Republic	..	18470	4.2	1.1	64.1	2.7	66	16	59	89	..
Iraq	..	..	..	..	20.1	2.1	44	12	75	45	..
Ireland	14710	..	4.7	4.1	3.6	0.4	105	..	58	..	..
Israel	15920	41178	6.4	3.2	5.5	2.7	87	..	..	99	..
Italy	19020	507926	1.0	0.7	57.2	0.2	81	..	67	..	..
Jamaica	1510	..	2.9	3.4	2.5	1.0	66	10	55	70	41.1
Japan	39640	..	1.0	0.8	125.2	0.3	..	3	78	95	..
Jordan	1510	1875	8.2	3.6	4.2	4.3	53	10	71	89	43.4
Kazakhstan	1330	..	-11.9	-11.8	16.6	-0.4	90	1	60	..	32.7
Kenya	280	2034	1.4	-1.3	26.7	2.6	25	23	28	49	57.5
Kiribati	920	..	..	-0.4	0.1	1.9	..	..	..	..	..
Korea, Dem. Rep.	..	..	..	..	23.9	1.8	..	..	61	..	..
Korea, Rep.	9700	80801	7.2	6.1	44.9	0.9	93	..	81	89	..
Kuwait	17390	13704	12.2	13.7	1.7	5.0	..	6	97	..	..
Kyrgyz Republic	700	..	-14.7	-15.1	4.5	0.3	..	..	39	75	..
Lao PDR	350	..	6.5	3.2	4.9	3.0	25	40	22	41	30.4
Latvia	2270	1433	-13.7	-13.3	2.5	-1.4	87	..	73	..	27.0
Lebanon	2660	3202	..	..	4.0	1.9	76	9	87	..	..
Lesotho	770	..	7.5	1.9	2.0	2.1	26	21	23	57	56.0
Liberia	..	..	..	..	2.7	2.4	..	20	45	..	..
Libya	..	..	..	..	5.4	3.5	97	5	86	30	..
Lithuania	1900	1520	-9.7	-9.7	3.7	-0.2	78	..	72	..	33.6
Luxembourg	41210	6217	..	-3.1	0.4	1.4	..	..	89	..	..
Macao	..	..	..	..	0.5	3.4	..	..	99	..	..
Macedonia, FYR	860	..	..	..	2.1	1.0	54	..	60	..	..
Madagascar	230	549	0.1	-2.8	13.7	3.1	18	32	27	32	43.4
Malawi	170	..	0.7	-2.2	9.8	2.7	4	28	14	54	..
Malaysia	3890	19605	8.7	5.9	20.1	2.4	59	23	54	90	48.4

Table A.6 (*continued*)

	Key Economic Indicators		*Average Annual Growth*		*Human Development*						
Country	*GNP/cap. 1995 (US$)*	*Central gov. exp. 1994–95 (US $ millions)*	*GDP 1990–95 (percent)*	*GNP/cap. 1990–95 (percent)*	*Population 1995 (millions)*	*Population growth rate 1995 (percent)*	*Gross sec. school enrollment mr 1985–95 (% of age group)*	*Child malnutrition mr 1985–95 (% of under-5 age group)*	*Urbanization mr 1985–95 (% of pop.)*	*Access to safe water mr 1985–95 (percent)*	*Gini index mr 1985–95 (percent)*
Maldives	990	117	..	3.9	0.3	3.2	49	39	33	..	..
Mali	250	..	2.5	-0.7	9.8	2.9	9	31	27	44	..
Malta	..	1064	..	..	0.4	1.0	88	..	89	..	..
Marshall Islands	..	..	..	..	..	..	..	..	..	..	..
Martinique	..	..	..	..	0.4	1.1	..	..	78	..	..
Mauritania	460	..	4.0	1.5	2.3	2.5	15	48	54	72	42.4
Mauritius	3380	915	4.9	3.4	1.1	1.4	59	15	41	100	..
Mayotte	..	..	..	..	..	..	..	..	..	..	..
Mexico	3320	63405	1.1	-1.2	91.8	1.9	58	19	75	87	50.3
Micronesia, Fed. Sts.	2010	..	..	..	0.1	2.2	..	..	28	..	..
Moldova	..	..	..	..	4.3	-0.1	69	..	52	..	34.4
Mongolia	310	206	-3.3	-5.9	2.5	2.1	82	12	61	54	..
Montserrat	..	..	..	..	0.0	0.4	..	..	14	..	..
Morocco	1110	..	1.2	-0.8	26.6	2.0	35	10	48	59	39.2
Mozambique	80	..	7.1	4.1	16.2	2.9	7	47	34	28	..
Myanmar	..	8034	5.7	..	45.1	1.7	..	31	26	39	..
Namibia	2000	..	3.8	0.8	1.5	2.7	55	26	37	57	..
Nepal	200	739	5.1	2.6	21.5	2.5	21	49	14	48	36.7
Netherlands	24000	201161	1.8	1.3	15.5	0.6	93	..	89	100	..
Netherlands Antilles	..	366	..	..	0.2	1.1	..	..	70	..	..
New Caledonia	..		..	..	0.2	1.9	..	..	62	..	..
New Zealand	14340	20605	3.6	2.3	3.6	1.4	104	..	86	..	..
Nicaragua	380	627	1.1	-1.7	4.4	3.1	41	12	63	57	50.3
Niger	220		0.5	-2.6	9.0	3.3	7	43	23	57	36.1
Nigeria	260		1.6	1.1	111.3	2.9	29	35	39	43	37.5
Norway	31250	50726	3.5	3.2	4.4	0.5	116	..	73	100	..
Oman	4820	5124	6.0	-0.8	2.2	5.5	61	14	13	56	..
Pakistan	460	13684	4.6	1.0	129.9	2.9	..	40	35	60	31.2
Panama	2750	1970	6.3	4.6	2.6	1.6	64	7	55	82	56.6
Papua New Guinea	1160	1612	9.3	6.0	4.3	2.3	12	30	16	31	..
Paraguay	1690		3.1	0.0	4.8	2.7	37	4	53	..	..
Peru	2310	10917	5.3	3.7	23.8	2.0	65	11	72	60	44.9
Philippines	1050		2.3	0.5	68.6	2.2	79	30	54	84	40.7
Poland	2790	51134	2.4	2.9	38.6	0.2	79	..	65	..	27.2
Portugal	9740	36990	0.8	0.7	9.9	0.1	..	..	36	..	..
Puerto Rico	..		3.0	..	3.7	1.1	..	..	73	..	..
Qatar	11600		..	-5.1	0.6	5.8	83	6	91	..	..
Reunion	..		..	..	0.7	1.7	..	..	68	..	..
Romania	1480	9607	-1.4	-1.2	22.7	-0.5	82	6	55	..	25.5
Russian Federation	2240	85762	-9.8	-10.2	148.2	-0.1	88	3	73	..	49.6
Rwanda	180		-12.8	-10.3	6.4	-2.8	10	29	6	..	28.9
Sao Tome & Principe	350		..	-1.5	0.1	2.5	..	17	47	..	..
Saudi Arabia	6810		1.7	-2.4	19.0	3.8	29	..	80	93	..
Senegal	600		1.9	-0.7	8.5	2.6	11	20	42	..	54.1
Seychelles	6620	269	..	2.6	0.1	1.6	104	6	65	..	..
Sierra Leone	180	179	-4.2	-4.1	4.2	0.8	..	29	36	..	..
Singapore	26730		8.7	6.4	3.0	1.9	84	14	100	100	..
Slovak Republic	2950		-2.8	-3.2	5.4	0.4	89	..	59	..	19.5
Slovenia	8200		..	..	2.0	-0.1	85	..	64	..	28.2
Solomon Islands	910		..	2.2	0.4	3.0	17	21	17	..	..
Somalia	..		..	..	9.5	4.1	..	39	26	..	..
South Africa	3160	40554	0.6	-1.1	41.5	2.2	77	9	51	..	58.4
Spain	13580		1.1	0.7	39.2	0.2	113	..	76	99	..
Sri Lanka	700	3649	4.8	3.7	18.1	1.2	74	38	22	57	30.1
St. Kitts and Nevis	5170	65	..	3.1	0.0	-0.5	103	..	46	..	..
St. Lucia	3370		..	3.1	0.2	0.9	..	..	46	..	..
St. Vincent & the Grenadines	2280	82	..	2.4	0.1	0.7	..	..	47	..	..

Country	*Key Economic Indicators* GNP/cap. 1995 (US$)	Central gov. exp. 1994–95 (US $ millions)	*Average Annual Growth* GDP 1990–95 (percent)	GNP/cap. 1990–95 (percent)	*Human Development* Population 1995 (millions)	Population growth rate 1995 (percent)	Gross sec. school enrollment mr 1985–95 (% of age group)	Child malnutrition mr 1985–95 (% of under-5 age group)	Urbanization mr 1985–95 (% of pop.)	Access to safe water mr 1985–95 (percent)	Gini index mr 1985–95 (percent)
Sudan	..		6.8	..	26.7	2.1	20	34	25	77	..
Suriname	880		..	0.3	0.4	0.4	35	..	50	..	..
Swaziland	1170		..	-1.4	0.9	2.5	51	10	31	..	..
Sweden	23750	102898	-0.1	-0.9	8.8	0.6	99	..	83	..	..
Switzerland	40630		0.1	-0.9	7.0	0.9	91	..	61	100	..
Syrian Arab Republic	1120	11759	7.4	4.3	14.1	3.0	47	..	52	87	..
Taiwan	12790		..	..	21.1	0.8	..	..	..	..	..
Tajikistan	340		-18.1	-20.3	5.8	1.6	100	..	32	..	..
Tanzania	120		3.2	0.4	29.6	3.0	..	29	24	49	38.1
Thailand	2740	26450	8.4	7.1	58.2	0.9	37	13	20	81	46.2
Togo	310		-3.4	-5.0	4.1	2.9	27	25	31	67	..
Tonga	1630		..	-0.3	0.1	3.1	..	..	41	..	..
Trinidad and Tobago	3770		1.0	0.0	1.3	0.8	76	7	67	82	..
Tunisia	1820		3.9	1.5	9.0	1.8	52	9	57	86	40.2
Turkey	2780	37518	3.2	1.5	61.1	1.6	61	10	69	92	..
Turkmenistan	920		-10.6	..	4.5	4.5	..	..	45	85	35.8
Turks & Caicos Isl.	..		..	..	..	..	..	..	..	..	..
Uganda	240		6.6	3.4	19.2	3.2	13	26	13	42	40.8
Ukraine	1630		-14.3	-14.4	51.6	-0.2	80	..	70	97	25.7
United Arab Emirates	17400	4277	..	-4.8	2.5	5.0	89	7	84	98	..
United Kingdom	18700	462387	1.4	1.3	58.5	0.3	92	..	89	100	..
United States	26980	1590000	2.6	1.5	263.1	1.0	97	..	76	90	..
Uruguay	5170	5576	4.0	3.9	3.2	0.6	81	4	90	34	..
Uzbekistan	970		-4.4	-6.4	22.8	2.1	94	4	41	..	..
Vanuatu	1200		..	-2.0	0.2	2.7	20	..	..	..	..
Venezuela	3020	10976	2.4	0.2	21.7	2.3	35	5	93	88	53.8
Viet Nam	..		8.3	..	73.5	2.0	35	45	21	38	35.7
Virgin Islands (UK)	..		..	..	..	..	..	..	..	..	..
Virgin Islands (US)	..		..	..	0.1	-0.5	..	..	49	..	..
West Bank	..		..	..	1.2	4.9	..	..	..	..	..
West Bank/Gaza Strip	..		..	..	..	..	..	..	..	..	..
Western Samoa	1120		..	-0.6	0.2	0.6	..	..	21	..	..
Yemen, Rep.	260		..	..	15.3	3.2	..	30	34	52	..
Yugoslavia, Fed. Republic	..		..	..	10.5	0.1	65	..	57	..	..
Zaire	120	468	..	..	43.8	3.2	24	34	29	25	..
Zambia	400	691	-0.2	-2.0	9.0	2.9	..	29	43	47	46.2
Zimbabwe	540		1.0	-1.7	11.0	2.4	45	16	32	74	56.8

Table A.6 (*continued*)

Country	Health Indicators: Life expectancy at birth 1995 (years)	% change in life expectancy 1980–95 (percent)	Infant mortality rate 1995 (per 1,000 live births)	Under-5 mortality rate 1995 (per 1,000 live births)	Adult mortality rate 1995 (per 1,000 adults, age 15–60)	Nutrition Indicators: Low birth weight 1985–95 mr 1985–95 (percent)	Anemia mr 1985–95 (% of pregnant women)	Obesity mr 1985–95 (% of children or adults)
Afghanistan	45	11	159	237	420	20	..	..
Albania	73	5	31	37	94	7	..	..
Algeria	69	18	34	42	155	9	42	..
Angola	47	13	124	209	450	19	29	..
Anguilla	..	..	..	..	..	..	..	..
Antigua and Barbuda	75	..	19	23	104	..	..	..
Argentina	73	5	22	27	130	6	26	7.0[a]
Armenia	71	-2	16	24	158	..	..	..
Aruba	..	..	..	..	..	..	..	..
Australia	77	4	6	8	85	..	..	..
Austria	77	6	6	7	106	6	..	..
Azerbaijan	70	3	25	31	161	..	..	..
Bahamas, The	73	8	15	18	119	..	12	..
Bahrain	73	7	19	23	139	..	..	..
Bangladesh	58	19	80	115	303	34	53	0.3[a]
Barbados	76	5	13	12	101	..	29	..
Belarus	70	-1	13	20	200	5	..	..
Belgium	77	5	8	10	101	6	..	..
Belize	74	..	37	46	147	..	65	..
Benin	50	7	96	156	436	10	41	..
Bermuda	..	..	..	..	..	..	..	..
Bhutan	..	..	..	175	..	..	81	..
Bolivia	60	16	70	96	264	12	54	..
Bosnia & Herzegovina	..	..	..	..	..	..	..	..
Botswana	52	-10	56	74	183	8	..	..
Brazil	67	7	45	57	152	11	33	5.4[a]
Brunei	75	6	9	11	113	..	..	..
Bulgaria	71	0	15	19	159	6	..	..
Burkina Faso	46	5	100	164	383	21	24	..
Burundi	46	-2	99	162	442	..	68	1.2[a]
Cambodia	53	36	109	158	334	..	..	..
Cameroon	57	14	57	86	377	13	44	..
Canada	78	5	6	8	95	6	..	..
Cape Verde	66	9	47	68	220	..	..	..
Cayman Islands	..	..	..	..	..	..	..	..
Central African Republic	49	6	98	160	456	15	67	4.8[a]
Chad	48	14	118	197	428	..	37	..
Channel Islands	78		7	9	89	..	..	..
Chile	75	8	12	15	119	7	13	6.6[a]
China	69	..	35	43	143	6	52	4.3[a]
Colombia	70	6	26	31	166	17	24	..
Comoros	56	11	89	143	320	..	..	..
Congo	51	3	90	144	359	16	..	3.4[b]
Costa Rica	77	6	13	16	92	..	28	..
Cote d'Ivoire	54	7	86	138	363	14	..	..
Croatia	74	5	16	18	127	8	..	..
Cuba	76	3	9	10	100	7	47	9.5[b]
Cyprus	78	4	8	11	88	..	..	..
Czech Republic	73	4	8	10	139	6	23	..
Denmark	75	1	6	7	119	5	..	..
Djibouti	50	13	109	181	412	..	40	..
Dominica	73	..	17	21	121	..	28	..
Dominican Republic	70	10	38	44	128	14	..	..
Ecuador	70	10	37	45	145	..	17	..
Egypt, Arab Republic	65	17	57	76	258	12	24	..
El Salvador	69	20	37	42	192	8	..	..
Equatorial Guinea	49	14	112	185	433	..	..	..

	Health Indicators					Nutrition Indicators		
Country	*Life expectancy at birth 1995 (years)*	*% change in life expectancy 1980–95 (percent)*	*Infant mortality rate 1995 (per 1,000 live births)*	*Under-5 mortality rate 1995 (per 1,000 live births)*	*Adult mortality rate 1995 (per 1,000 adults, age 15–60)*	*Low birth weight 1985–95 mr 1985–95 (percent)*	*Anemia mr 1985–95 (% of pregnant women)*	*Obesity mr 1985–95 (% of children or adults)*
Eritrea	50	13	132	196	385	..	..	..
Estonia	70	2	14	16	189	..	..	..
Ethiopia	49	19	113	188	397	16	42	..
Fiji	72	6	21	25	133	..	..	..
Finland	76	5	5	5	107	5	..	..
France	78	5	6	9	107	..	..	..
French Guiana	..	..	..	..	..	..	..	..
French Polynesia	70		17	24	185	..	..	..
Gabon	54	13	90	145	354	10	..	..
Gambia, The	46	15	127	213	465	10	80	..
Gaza Strip	..	..	31	51	125	..	..	..
Georgia	73	3	18	21	133	..	..	..
Germany	76	5	6	7	108	..	..	..
Ghana	59	12	74	116	287	17	..	3.2[b]
Greece	78	5	8	10	87	9	..	..
Grenada	..	..	..	32	..	..	..	..
Guadeloupe	75	6	11	14	112	..	..	..
Guam	73	..	9	12	139	..	..	..
Guatemala	65	13	45	58	206	14	..	2.8[a]
Guinea	45	12	129	220	498	21	..	..
Guinea-Bissau	43	13	137	233	578	20	74	..
Guyana	64	5	61	82	200	..	71	2.3[a]
Haiti	56	8	73	101	360	15	..	..
Honduras	67	11	46	59	138	..	14	1.8[a]
Hong Kong	79	6	5	6	83	..	..	..
Hungary	70	0	11	14	234	9	..	..
Iceland	79	3	4	6	80	..	..	..
India	62	15	69	95	224	33	88	0.5[b]
Indonesia	64	17	52	75	233	14	64	..
Iran, Islamic Republic	68	14	46	59	154	12	..	..
Iraq	61	-2	111	145	162	15	18	..
Ireland	76	5	6	7	99	4	..	..
Israel	77	6	8	9	85	..	..	..
Italy	78	5	7	8	91	..	..	..
Jamaica	74	5	13	15	117	11	40	..
Japan	80	5	4	6	74	6	..	..
Jordan	70	..	31	33	145	7	..	..
Kazakhstan	69	3	27	35	208	..	11	15.0[a]
Kenya	59	7	59	90	329	16	35	2.4[b]
Kiribati	58	..	56	75	..	..	..	..
Korea, Dem. Rep.	70	5	27	32	159	..	..	..
Korea, Rep.	72	8	10	14	163	4	..	..
Kuwait	76	8	11	14	97	..	40	..
Kyrgyz Republic	68	3	30	42	198	..	..	..
Lao PDR	52	17	92	147	410	18	..	0.7[b]
Latvia	69	-1	16	20	215	..	..	..
Lebanon	69	6	32	40	163	..	..	..
Lesotho	58	10	77	121	302	11	7	..
Liberia	45	-11	177	239	225	..	78	..
Libya	65	13	62	75	190	5	..	..
Lithuania	69	-2	14	19	201	..	..	..
Luxembourg	76	5	6	9	108	..	..	..
Macao	77	17	7	9	..	..	..	..
Macedonia, FYR	73	..	23	31	118	..	..	..
Madagascar	58	14	90	127	415	10	..	..
Malawi	44	-1	133	225	520	20	55	..
Malaysia	71	7	12	14	146	8	56	..

Table A.6 (*continued*)

	Health Indicators					Nutrition Indicators		
Country	*Life expectancy at birth 1995 (years)*	*% change in life expectancy 1980–95 (percent)*	*Infant mortality rate 1995 (per 1,000 live births)*	*Under-5 mortality rate 1995 (per 1,000 live births)*	*Adult mortality rate 1995 (per 1,000 adults, age 15–60)*	*Low birth weight 1985–95 mr 1985–95 (percent)*	*Anemia mr 1985–95 (% of pregnant women)*	*Obesity mr 1985–95 (% of children or adults)*
Maldives	63	14	53	70	235	..	20	..
Mali	49	18	124	192	369	17	58	0.5[a]
Malta	77	5	9	11	95	..	..	..
Marshall Islands	..	..	..	..	..	..	..	..
Martinique	77	5	8	12	100	..	..	..
Mauritania	53	13	97	158	432	11	..	..
Mauritius	71	8	16	20	169	8	29	5.6[b]
Mayotte	..	..	..	..	..	..	..	..
Mexico	71	7	33	41	125	12	14	..
Micronesia, Fed. Sts.	64	..	33	40	265	..	..	..
Moldova	69	5	22	26	202	..	50	..
Mongolia	65	13	56	74	201	10	45	..
Montserrat	73	..	25	31	122	..	..	..
Morocco	66	14	56	75	188	9	45	5.2[a]
Mozambique	46	6	114	190	385	20	58	..
Myanmar	59	13	84	119	280	16	58	..
Namibia	56	6	62	78	330	12	16	..
Nepal	56	17	92	131	340	26	65	..
Netherlands	78	3	6	8	88	..	..	..
Netherlands Antilles	77	8	11	14	88	..	..	..
New Caledonia	73	12	16	19	125	..	..	..
New Zealand	76	4	7	9	104	6	..	..
Nicaragua	67	15	47	61	153	15	36	..
Niger	47	12	120	..	455	15	41	..
Nigeria	52	14	81	176	414	16	55	..
Norway	78	3	5	8	89	5	..	..
Oman	70	19	18	22	167	10	54	..
Pakistan	63	14	91	127	218	25	37	..
Panama	74	5	23	28	113	..	..	..
Papua New Guinea	57	12	65	95	355	23	13	1.6[a]
Paraguay	69	3	41	52	133	5	29	..
Peru	66	13	48	62	184	11	53	9.0[b]
Philippines	66	8	40	53	222	..	48	0.9[a]
Poland	72	1	14	16	136	8	16	..
Portugal	75	5	7	11	120	5	..	..
Puerto Rico	76	3	11	15	104	..	..	..
Qatar	72	8	19	22	139	..	..	..
Reunion	74	8	8	10	131	..	..	..
Romania	70	0	23	29	195	..	31	..
Russian Federation	65	-3	18	21	322	..	30	..
Rwanda	38	-16	135	200	502	17	..	..
Sao Tome & Principe	69	..	61	78	117	..	..	..
Saudi Arabia	70	15	21	31	165	..	..	..
Senegal	50	11	63	97	529	11	26	3.7[b]
Seychelles	72	..	15	19	147	..	..	..
Sierra Leone	36	2	182	236	529	17	..	..
Singapore	76	7	4	6	103	7	..	..
Slovak Republic	72	2	11	15	157	6	..	..
Slovenia	74	5	7	8	134	6	..	..
Solomon Islands	62	..	41	52	284	..	..	..
Somalia	48	13	129	218	356	16	78	..
South Africa	64	13	51	67	..	..	37	..
Spain	77	2	7	9	99	..	..	..
Sri Lanka	73	7	16	19	140	17	39	0.1[a]
St. Kitts and Nevis	69	..	31	38	169	..	..	..
St. Lucia	71	..	17	21	163	..	..	..
St. Vincent & the Grenadines	72	..	19	22	140	..	..	..

Country	Health Indicators: Life expectancy at birth 1995 (years)	% change in life expectancy 1980–95 (percent)	Infant mortality rate 1995 (per 1,000 live births)	Under-5 mortality rate 1995 (per 1,000 live births)	Adult mortality rate 1995 (per 1,000 adults, age 15–60)	Nutrition Indicators: Low birth weight 1985–95 mr 1985–95 (percent)	Anemia mr 1985–95 (% of pregnant women)	Obesity mr 1985–95 (% of children or adults)
Sudan	53	11	78	109	411	15	36	..
Suriname	70	7	34	41	155	..	..	..
Swaziland	59	15	70	96	220	..	..	..
Sweden	79	4	4	5	81	5	..	..
Switzerland	79	4	6	7	87	5	..	..
Syrian Arab Republic	68	11	33	40	186	8	..	..
Taiwan	76	4	6	7	121	..	..	..
Tajikistan	66	0	42	61	199	..	50	..
Tanzania	51	2	83	133	451	14	..	..
Thailand	69	9	35	42	159	13	57	1.3[a]
Togo	51	3	89	128	344	20	48	2.5[a]
Tonga	69	..	19	23	193	..	..	..
Trinidad and Tobago	72	6	14	18	150	13	53	3.3[a]
Tunisia	69	11	40	50	160	10	..	3.8[a]
Turkey	68	11	49	63	135	8	..	..
Turkmenistan	..	..	46	65	186	..	..	..
Turks & Caicos Isl.	..	..	..	..	..	..	..	..
Uganda	44	-9	98	160	590	..	30	2.4[a]
Ukraine	69	-1	15	21	203	5	..	..
United Arab Emirates	75	10	16	19	107	..	46	..
United Kingdom	77	4	6	7	95	..	..	..
United States	77	4	8	10	123	7	..	..
Uruguay	73	4	18	21	129	..	20	..
Uzbekistan	..	..	30	48	155	..	..	7.8[a]
Vanuatu	64	..	42	51	247	..	..	..
Venezuela	72	6	23	25	133	10	29	3.3[a]
Viet Nam	68	7	41	49	171	17	52.3	..
Virgin Islands (UK)	..	..	..	..	..	..	..	..
Virgin Islands (US)	76	..	19	23	98	..	..	..
West Bank	..	..	27	45	126	..	..	..
West Bank/Gaza Strip	..	..	..	..	..	..	..	..
Western Samoa	69	9	23	27	190	..	..	..
Yemen, Rep.	53	11	101	145	358	19	..	..
Yugoslavia, Fed. Republic	72	3	18	22	134	..	..	..
Zaire	..	..	..	144	..	15	76	..
Zambia	46	-8	109	180	514	13	34	5.7[b]
Zimbabwe	58	5	55	83	392	14	..	4.4[a]

a. Data for adults.
b. Data for children.

Note: .. indicates data not available.

Table A.6 (*continued*)

Country	Reproductive Health Indicators: Adolescent fertility rate 1995 (per 1,000 women, age 15–19)	Total fertility rate 1995 (per woman, age 15–49)	Total fertility change 1980–95 (percent)	Unwanted fertility rate 1990–95 (per woman, age 15–49)	Maternal mortality rate 1990–95 (per 100,000 live births)	Future Challenges: Tuberculosis incidence 1995 (per 100,000 population)	Adult HIV/AIDS prevalence 1994 (percent)	Smoking prevalence (% of adults): Male	Smoking prevalence (% of adults): Female
Afghanistan	153	6.9	-2	..	1700	278	0.0	..	..
Albania	26	2.6	-27	..	23	40	0.0	50	8
Algeria	17	3.6	-47	..	140	53	0.1	53	10
Angola	218	6.9	1	..	1500	225	1.0	..	..
Anguilla	..	..	..	..	..	20	..	..	..
Antigua and Barbuda	57	1.7	-21	..	..	20	..	..	..
Argentina	62	2.7	-17	..	140	50	0.4	40	23
Armenia	50	1.8	-22	..	35	40	0.0	..	..
Aruba	..	..	..	..	..	..	..	..	..
Australia	31	1.9	-2	..	9	6	0.1	29	21
Austria	23	1.5	-10	..	10	20	0.2	42	27
Azerbaijan	33	2.3	-29	..	29	47	0.0	..	..
Bahamas, The	56	2.0	-41	..	100	30	3.9	19	4
Bahrain	27	3.2	-39	..	60	25	0.2	24	6
Bangladesh	116	3.5	-43	1.3	887	220	0.0	60	15
Barbados	50	1.8	-12	..	43	20	2.8	..	..
Belarus	39	1.4	-31	..	25	50	0.0	..	..
Belgium	11	1.6	-3	..	10	16	0.2	31	19
Belize	92	3.9	..	..	..	40	2.0	..	..
Benin	127	6.1	-7	..	990	135	1.2	..	..
Bermuda	..	..	..	..	..	20	..	..	..
Bhutan	67	..	..	..	..	90	0.0	..	..
Bolivia	82	4.6	-17	1.9	373	335	0.1	50	21
Bosnia & Herzegovina	28	..	..	..	..	80	0.0	..	..
Botswana	106	4.4	-34	..	220	400	18.0	21	..
Brazil	37	2.4	-38	..	200	80	0.7	40	25
Brunei	28	3.0	-28	..	60	70	0.2	..	..
Bulgaria	60	1.2	-40	..	20	40	0.0	49	17
Burkina Faso	149	6.8	-10	0.9	939	289	6.7	..	..
Burundi	66	6.5	-4	..	1327	367	2.7	..	..
Cambodia	108	4.7	3	..	900	235	1.9	80	10
Cameroon	136	5.7	-12	0.6	550	194	3.0	..	..
Canada	25	1.7	-3	..	6	8	0.2	31	29
Cape Verde	26	4.0	-38	..	..	100	..	..	..
Cayman Islands	..	..	..	..	..	20	..	..	..
Central African Republic	145	5.1	-11	..	649	139	5.8	..	..
Chad	183	5.9	0	..	1594	167	2.7	..	..
Channel Islands	21	1.7	18	..	..	..	..	..	..
Chile	48	2.4	-18	..	65	67	0.1	38	25
China	17	1.9	-24	..	115	85	0.0	63	4
Colombia	80	2.8	-27	0.8	107	67	0.2	35	19
Comoros	131	6.0	..	..	950	150	0.1	..	..
Congo	140	6.1	-1	..	822	250	7.2	..	..
Costa Rica	67	2.9	-22	..	55	15	0.5	35	20
Cote d'Ivoire	136	5.4	-28	1.0	887	196	6.8	..	..
Croatia	28	1.5	..	..	10	65	0.0	37	38
Cuba	68	1.7	-16	..	36	20	0.0	39	25
Cyprus	34	2.2	-11	..	5	15	0.3	43	7
Czech Republic	34	1.3	-38	..	12	25	0.0	43	31
Denmark	18	1.8	16	..	9	12	0.2	37	37
Djibouti	171	5.8	-12	..	570	600	3.0	..	..
Dominica	47	2.4	..	..	..	20	..	..	..
Dominican Republic	53	2.9	-31	..	110	110	1.0	66	14
Ecuador	68	3.3	-35	..	150	166	0.3	52	28
Egypt, Arab Republic	56	3.5	-32	1.0	170	78	0.0	40	2
El Salvador	91	3.7	-31	..	300	110	0.6	38	12
Equatorial Guinea	182	5.9	3	..	820	150	1.1	..	..

Country	*Reproductive Health Indicators*					*Future Challenges*			
	Adolescent fertility rate 1995 (per 1,000 women, age 15–19)	*Total fertility rate 1995 (per woman, age 15–49)*	*Total fertility change 1980–95 (percent)*	*Unwanted fertility rate 1990–95 (per woman, age 15–49)*	*Maternal mortality rate 1990–95 (per 100,000 live births)*	*Tuberculosis incidence 1995 (per 100,000 population)*	*Adult HIV/AIDS prevalence 1994 (percent)*	*Smoking prevalence (% of adults)*	
								Male	*Female*
Eritrea	125	5.8	..	..	1400	155	3.2	..	..
Estonia	36	1.3	-35	..	41	60	0.0	52	24
Ethiopia	164	7.0	8	..	1528	155	2.5	..	..
Fiji	43	2.8	-22	..	90	40	0.0	59	31
Finland	20	1.8	11	..	11	15	0.0	27	19
France	17	1.7	-13	..	15	20	0.3	40	27
French Guiana	..	..	..	..	..	100	..	..	..
French Polynesia	51	3.0	..	..	..	60	..	..	..
Gabon	150	5.2	17	..	483	100	2.3	..	..
Gambia, The	167	5.3	-18	..	1050	166	2.1	..	..
Gaza Strip	119	7.1	3	..	..	..	..	..	..
Georgia	40	..	..	..	55	70	0.0	45	35
Germany	14	1.2	-21	..	22	18	0.1	37	22
Ghana	109	5.2	-20	..	742	222	2.3	10	1
Greece	19	1.4	-39	..	10	12	0.1	46	28
Grenada	59	..	..	..	..	20	..	..	..
Guadeloupe	34	2.1	-25	..	..	20	..	..	..
Guam	58	2.7	..	..	..	80	..	..	..
Guatemala	106	4.8	-23	1.1	464	110	0.4	38	18
Guinea	213	6.5	7	..	880	166	0.6	40	2
Guinea-Bissau	186	6.0	0	..	910	220	3.1	..	..
Guyana	56	2.4	-32	..	..	50	1.3	..	..
Haiti	70	4.5	-24	1.8	600	333	4.4	..	..
Honduras	112	4.7	-28	..	220	133	1.6	36	11
Hong Kong	13	1.2	-40	..	7	140	0.1	..	..
Hungary	31	1.6	-18	..	10	50	0.1	44	27
Iceland	29	2.1	-14	..	0	10	0.1	31	28
India	81	3.2	-35	0.8	437	220	0.4	40	3
Indonesia	57	2.7	-39	0.5	390	220	0.0	53	4
Iran, Islamic Republic	80	4.6	-26	..	120	50	0.0	..	..
Iraq	61	5.5	-15	..	310	150	0.0	40	5
Ireland	23	1.9	-42	..	10	18	0.1	29	28
Israel	28	2.4	-26	..	7	12	0.1	45	30
Italy	14	1.2	-29	..	12	25	0.3	38	26
Jamaica	67	2.5	-35	..	120	10	0.9	43	13
Japan	6	1.5	-14	..	18	42	0.0	59	15
Jordan	43	4.8	-30	..	132	14	0.0	48	9
Kazakhstan	40	2.3	-22	..	53	77	0.0	..	..
Kenya	95	4.8	-39	2.0	650	140	8.3	52	7
Kiribati	54	3.8	-17	..	..	400	..	..	..
Korea, Dem. Rep.	30	2.2	-28	..	48	162	0.0	..	..
Korea, Rep.	8	1.8	-33	..	30	162	0.0	68	7
Kuwait	45	3.0	-44	..	18	40	0.1	52	12
Kyrgyz Republic	44	3.3	-20	..	80	68	0.0	48	15
Lao PDR	59	6.5	-2	..	660	235	0.0	41	15
Latvia	34	1.3	-38	..	40	70	0.0	67	12
Lebanon	43	2.9	-29	..	300	35	0.1	..	..
Lesotho	55	4.7	-17	..	598	250	3.1	38	1
Liberia	211	6.6	-3	..	560	100	1.3	..	..
Libya	106	6.1	-16	..	220	12	0.1	..	..
Lithuania	34	1.5	-24	..	16	82	0.0	52	10
Luxembourg	16	1.7	12	..	0	10	0.1	32	26
Macao	15	1.9	..	..	..	100	..	..	..
Macedonia, FYR	38	2.2	-14	..	12	60	0.0	..	..
Madagascar	145	5.9	-10	0.9	660	310	0.1	29	28
Malawi	151	6.6	-13	1.0	620	173	13.6	..	..
Malaysia	30	3.4	-19		34	67	0.3	41	4

Table A.6 (*continued*)

Country	Reproductive Health Indicators: Adolescent fertility rate 1995 (per 1,000 women, age 15–19)	Total fertility rate 1995 (per woman, age 15–49)	Total fertility change 1980–95 (percent)	Unwanted fertility rate 1990–95 (per woman, age 15–49)	Maternal mortality rate 1990–95 (per 100,000 live births)	Future Challenges: Tuberculosis incidence 1995 (per 100,000 population)	Adult HIV/AIDS prevalence 1994 (percent)	Smoking prevalence (% of adults): Male	Smoking prevalence (% of adults): Female
Maldives	76	6.7	-4	..	..	120	0.1	..	..
Mali	190	6.9	-4	0.7	1249	289	1.3	..	..
Malta	13	1.9	-8	..	0	10	0.1	40	18
Marshall Islands	..	..	..	..	..	150	..	..	..
Martinique	32	2.0	-15	..	..	20	..	..	..
Mauritania	123	5.2	-17	..	800	220	0.7	..	..
Mauritius	42	2.2	-20	..	112	50	0.1	47	4
Mayotte	..	..	..	..	..	..	..	..	..
Mexico	57	3.0	-34	..	110	60	0.4	38	14
Micronesia, Fed. Sts.	51	4.6	..	..	..	60	..	..	..
Moldova	46	2.0	-18	..	34	70	0.0	..	..
Mongolia	45	3.4	-37	..	240	100	0.0	40	7
Montserrat	62	2.3	..	..	..	20	..	..	..
Morocco	38	3.5	-37	1.4	372	125	0.0	40	9
Mozambique	122	6.3	-3	..	1512	189	5.8	..	..
Myanmar	30	3.5	-32	..	518	189	1.5	..	..
Namibia	130	5.0	-15	..	370	400	6.5	..	..
Nepal	82	5.3	-17	..	515	167	0.1	..	..
Netherlands	8	1.6	-1	..	12	13	0.0	36	29
Netherlands Antilles	33	2.1	-11	..	..	20	..	..	..
New Caledonia	47	2.5	-34	..	..	90	..	..	..
New Zealand	43	2.1	-1	..	25	10	0.1	24	22
Nicaragua	136	4.2	-32	..	160	110	0.1	..	..
Niger	222	7.4	0	0.3	593	144	1.0	41	26
Nigeria	120	5.6	-19	1.0	1000	222	2.2	24	7
Norway	22	1.9	9	..	6	8	0.1	36	36
Oman	123	7.1	-29	..	190	20	0.1	..	..
Pakistan	107	5.3	-24	1.2	340	150	0.1	27	4
Panama	61	2.7	-29	..	55	90	0.6	56	20
Papua New Guinea	44	4.8	-15	..	930	275	0.2	46	28
Paraguay	72	4.1	-16	..	180	166	0.1	24	6
Peru	52	3.2	-31	1.5	280	250	0.2	41	13
Philippines	47	3.8	-23	1.2	208	400	0.1	43	8
Poland	28	1.6	-29	..	10	50	0.1	51	29
Portugal	23	1.4	-34	..	15	60	0.2	38	15
Puerto Rico	48	2.1	-17	..	21	8	..	..	..
Qatar	40	3.9	-32	..	..	50	0.1	..	..
Reunion	51	2.2	-29	..	..	..	0.0	..	..
Romania	34	1.4	-42	..	48	120	0.0	43	15
Russian Federation	31	1.4	-26	..	52	99	0.0	67	30
Rwanda	65	6.3	-24	2.0	1512	260	7.2	..	..
Sao Tome & Principe	149	4.8	..	..	..	100	..	..	..
Saudi Arabia	61	6.3	-14	..	18	22	0.0	53	
Senegal	118	5.8	-14	0.9	510	166	1.4	48	35
Seychelles	51	2.5	..	..	..	40	..	..	..
Sierra Leone	203	6.5	0	..	800	167	3.0	..	..
Singapore	13	1.7	-2	..	10	82	0.1	32	3
Slovak Republic	35	1.5	-34	..	8	40	0.0	43	26
Slovenia	19	1.3	-38	..	5	35	0.0	35	23
Solomon Islands	94	5.2	-23	..	..	120	..	..	..
Somalia	191	7.0	0	..	1600	222	0.3	..	..
South Africa	68	3.9	-21	..	404	250	3.2	52	17
Spain	11	1.2	-47	..	7	49	0.6	48	25
Sri Lanka	33	2.3	-34	..	30	167	0.1	55	1
St. Kitts and Nevis	68	2.4	..	..	..	25	..	..	..
St. Lucia	84	3.0	-32	..	..	20	..	..	..
St. Vincent & the Grenadines	52	2.3	..	..	..	25	..	..	..

Country	Reproductive Health Indicators					Future Challenges			
	Adolescent fertility rate 1995 (per 1,000 women, age 15–19)	*Total fertility rate 1995 (per woman, age 15–49)*	*Total fertility change 1980–95 (percent)*	*Unwanted fertility rate 1990–95 (per woman, age 15–49)*	*Maternal mortality rate 1990–95 (per 100,000 live births)*	*Tuberculosis incidence 1995 (per 100,000 population)*	*Adult HIV/AIDS prevalence 1994 (percent)*	*Smoking prevalence (% of adults)* Male	Female
Sudan	84	4.8	-27	1.5	660	211	1.0	..	..
Suriname	52	2.6	-39	..	..	100	1.2	..	..
Swaziland	111	4.7	-26	..	560	200	3.8	33	8
Sweden	20	1.7	4	..	7	7	0.1	22	24
Switzerland	7	1.5	-5	..	6	18	0.3	36	26
Syrian Arab Republic	89	4.9	-34	..	179	58	0.0	..	..
Taiwan	24	1.8	-33	..	..	..	..	..	..
Tajikistan	48	4.2	-26	..	39	133	0.0	..	..
Tanzania	123	5.8	-14	0.7	748	187	6.4	..	..
Thailand	18	1.8	-49	..	200	173	2.1	49	4
Togo	124	6.4	-2	..	626	244	8.5	..	..
Tonga	32	3.3	-32	..	..	40	..	65	14
Trinidad and Tobago	46	2.1	-35	..	90	20	0.9	42	8
Tunisia	32	3.0	-43	..	139	55	0.0	58	6
Turkey	44	2.7	-37	0.9	183	57	0.0	63	24
Turkmenistan	26	3.8	-24	..	43	72	0.0	27	1
Turks & Caicos Isl.	..	..	..	..	..	20	..	..	..
Uganda	193	6.8	-6	1.3	506	300	14.5	10	0
Ukraine	48	1.5	-25	..	33	50	0.0	50	47
United Arab Emirates	58	3.6	-33	..	33	30	0.2	..	..
United Kingdom	30	1.7	-10	..	20	12	0.1	28	26
United States	60	2.1	12	..	12	10	0.5	28	23
Uruguay	47	2.2	-18	..	85	20	0.3	41	27
Uzbekistan	43	3.7	-23	..	43	55	0.0	49	9
Vanuatu	55	5.0	..	..	280	120	..	..	..
Venezuela	60	3.1	-26	..	200	44	0.3	..	..
Viet Nam	42	3.1	-39	..	105	166	0.1	73	4
Virgin Islands (UK)	..	..	..	..	..	20	..	..	..
Virgin Islands (US)	74	2.4	..	..	..	20	..	..	..
West Bank	90	5.6	..	..	..	..	..	..	..
West Bank/Gaza Strip	..	..	..	..	..	..	..	..	..
Western Samoa	42	4.3	..	..	35	30	..	..	..
Yemen, Rep.	141	7.4	-6	1.7	1471	96	0.0	..	..
Yugoslavia, Fed. Republic	41	1.9	-20	..	..	50	0.1	52	31
Zaire	221	..	..	..	870	333	3.7	..	..
Zambia	122	5.7	-19	..	230	345	17.1	39	7
Zimbabwe	68	3.9	-43	0.8	570	207	17.4	36	15

.. = Data not available.

Table A.6 (*continued*)

	Health Services Indicators				Health Finance Indicators					
Country	*In-patient beds per 1,000 pop. mr 1990–95*	*Physicians per 1,000 pop. mr 1990–95*	*Access to health services, % mr 1990–95*	*Immunization coverage, measles, % mr 1990–95*	*Year*	*Total health expenditures % of GDP*	*Health expenditures (public) % of GDP*	*Health expenditures (public) per cap. US$*	*Total health expenditures per cap. US$*	*Total health expenditures PPP$*
Afghanistan	0.2	0.1	..	19	..	..	..	..	..	..
Albania	3.2	1.4	..	91	1995	..	2.7	16	..	..
Algeria	2.1	0.8	..	69	1993	4.6	3.3	61	85	247
Angola	1.3	0.0	24	32	1991	..	4.0	60	..	..
Anguilla	..	1.1	..	..	1994	4.7	2.2	..	..	..
Antigua and Barbuda	6.1	0.9	..	..	1994	6.4	3.9	296	484	..
Argentina	4.6	2.7	..	76	1994	10.6	4.3	354	877	932
Armenia	8.4	3.1	..	95	1995	7.8	3.1	11	27	140
Aruba	..	1.1	..	..	..	..	..	..	..	..
Australia	8.9	2.2	100	86	1994	8.4	5.8	1079	1575	1725
Austria	9.3	2.6	100	60	1994	9.7	6.2	1524	2404	2147
Azerbaijan	10.0	3.9	..	91	1995	7.5	1.4	4	24	96
Bahamas, The	3.9	1.4	..	88	1994	4.4	2.6	321	546	708
Bahrain	..	1.3	..	90	1991	5.7	..	..	473	280
Bangladesh	0.3	0.2	74	96	1995	2.4	1.2	3	6	35
Barbados	8.4	1.1	..	52	1994	6.9	4.4	290	449	790
Belarus	11.6	4.1	100	96	1995	6.4	5.3	1517	1829	280
Belgium	7.6	3.7	100	70	1995	8.0	7.0	1866	2125	1784
Belize	2.8	0.5	..	83	1994	8.2	6.1	161	214	472
Benin	0.2	0.1	42	72	1994	..	1.7	5	20	83
Bermuda	..	1.2	..	..	1994	3.5	0.5	165	1064	..
Bhutan	1.6	0.2	..	58	1995	..	2.2	10	..	..
Bolivia	1.4	0.5	..	83	1994	5.0	2.7	20	38	138
Bosnia & Herzegovina	1.8	0.5	..	57	..	..	..	..	..	..
Botswana	1.6	..	86	68	1992	3.1	1.9	52	81	171
Brazil	3.0	1.4	..	78	1994	7.4	2.7	95	261	428
Brunei	..	0.7	..	92	1991	..	1.8	269	..	..
Bulgaria	10.6	3.5	100	93	1992	6.9	5.5	56	70	296
Burkina Faso	0.3	..	..	55	1992	5.5	2.3	7	17	43
Burundi	0.7	0.1	80	44	1995	..	0.9	2	..	..
Cambodia	2.1	0.1	..	75	1994	7.2	0.7	2	18	..
Cameroon	2.6	0.1	15	31	1994	1.4	1.0	5	7	33
Canada	6.0	2.2	99	98	1994	9.8	7.0	1304	1814	2213
Cape Verde	1.6	0.2	..	95	1994	..	3.5	32	..	..
Cayman Islands	3.0	1.7	..	..	1994	4.8	2.8	1082	1856	..
Central African Republic	0.9	0.0	13	70	1995	..	1.9	6	..	..
Chad	0.7	..	26	24	1995	..	2.5	4	9	29
Channel Islands	..	..	..	..	..	..	..	..	..	..
Chile	3.1	1.1	95	93	1994	6.5	2.5	93	241	652
China	2.4	1.6	..	89	1993	3.8	1.8	9	19	98
Colombia	1.4	1.1	87	77	1994	7.4	3.0	55	138	487
Comoros	2.8	0.1	..	60	1993	1.2	0.9	5	7	18
Congo	3.3	0.3	..	39	1992	6.8	3.6	44	83	183
Costa Rica	2.5	1.3	97	94	1994	8.5	6.3	158	214	536
Cote d'Ivoire	0.8	0.1	60	57	1995	3.4	1.4	10	25	71
Croatia	5.9	2.0	..	90	1994	10.1	8.5	253	302	..
Cuba	5.4	3.6	100	100	1994	..	7.9	..	..	..
Cyprus	..	1.8	..	83	1993	4.6	..	..	414	..
Czech Republic	9.2	3.0	..	96	1995	9.6	7.7	336	417	970
Denmark	5.0	2.9	100	88	1994	6.6	5.5	1537	2191	1497
Djibouti	2.6	0.2	..	68	..	..	..	..	..	..
Dominica	2.6	0.5	..	99	..	..	..	..	..	..
Dominican Republic	2.0	1.1	..	100	1994	5.3	2.0	27	71	220
Ecuador	1.6	1.5	80	100	1994	5.3	2.0	30	78	253
Egypt, Arab Republic	1.9	1.8	99	82	1990	5.3	2.2	23	56	191
El Salvador	1.5	0.8	..	94	1994	5.0	1.2	18	74	132
Equatorial Guinea	..	0.3	..	70	1990	7.2	5.8	22	27	..

Country	Health Services Indicators				Health Finance Indicators					
	In-patient beds per 1,000 pop. mr 1990–95	Physicians per 1,000 pop. mr 1990–95	Access to health services, % mr 1990–95	Immunization coverage, measles, % mr 1990–95	Year	Total health expenditures % of GDP	Health expenditures (public) % of GDP	Health expenditures (public) per cap. US$	Total health expenditures per cap. US$	Total health expenditures PPP$
Eritrea	..	..	..	45	1994	2.0	1.1	..	..	..
Estonia	8.0	3.1	..	81	1995	..	6.3	91	..	..
Ethiopia	0.2	..	55	54	1994	..	1.1	1	..	..
Fiji	..	0.6	..	93	1992	3.4	2.0	42	70	176
Finland	10.1	2.7	100	98	1994	8.3	6.2	1196	1591	1585
France	9.0	2.8	..	76	1995	9.8	7.7	1755	2599	2139
French Guiana	..	1.3	..	..	..	..	..	..	..	..
French Polynesia	..	..	..	..	..	..	..	..	..	..
Gabon	3.3	..	87	50	1994	..	0.6	19	..	..
Gambia, The	0.6	..	..	88	1994	..	1.9	6	..	..
Gaza Strip	..	..	..	..	..	..	..	..	..	..
Georgia	8.2	4.1	..	63	1995	..	0.8	3	..	..
Germany	9.7	3.3	..	75	1995	9.6	7.0	1751	2823	1976
Ghana	1.5	..	25	68	1995	..	1.3	3	..	..
Greece	5.1	4.0	..	70	1993	5.7	4.3	305	474	759
Grenada	8.1	0.6	..	..	..	..	..	..	..	..
Guadeloupe	..	1.4	..	..	..	..	..	..	..	..
Guam	..	..	..	..	..	..	..	..	..	..
Guatemala	1.1	0.8	60	84	1994	2.7	0.9	12	33	92
Guinea	0.6	0.1	45	69	1994	..	0.9	5	..	..
Guinea-Bissau	1.5	..	80	68	1994	..	1.1	3	..	..
Guyana	2.8	0.1	..	90	..	..	..	..	..	..
Haiti	0.8	0.1	45	24	1994	3.6	1.3	3	8	35
Honduras	1.0	0.4	62	90	1994	5.6	2.8	17	34	121
Hong Kong	4.3	1.3	..	42	1994	4.3	1.9	411	944	1036
Hungary	9.9	3.4	..	100	1994	7.3	6.8	275	295	496
Iceland	15.9	3.0	..	98	1995	8.1	6.9	1596	2144	1767
India	0.8	..	..	84	1992	5.6	1.2	2	8	68
Indonesia	0.7	0.2	43	89	1994	1.5	0.7	7	14	63
Iran, Islamic Republic	1.4	..	73	95	1990	4.8	2.8	271	467	239
Iraq	1.7	0.2	98	95	..	..	..	..	..	..
Ireland	5.0	2.0	..	78	1994	7.9	6.0	875	1151	1451
Israel	3.2	..	100	94	1990	4.2	2.1	249	546	665
Italy	6.7	1.7	..	50	1995	7.7	5.4	1051	1471	1605
Jamaica	2.1	0.5	..	82	1994	5.4	3.0	51	91	212
Japan	15.5	1.8	100	68	1994	7.0	5.5	2066	2947	1659
Jordan	1.6	1.6	90	92	1994	7.9	3.7	55	118	347
Kazakhstan	11.6	3.6	..	72	1994	..	2.2	15	..	..
Kenya	1.7	0.0	..	73	1992	2.5	1.6	5	8	34
Kiribati	4.3	0.2	..	89	1990	..	8.9	158	..	..
Korea, Dem. Rep.	..	..	100	98	..	..	..	..	..	..
Korea, Rep.	4.1	1.2	100	92	1992	5.4	1.8	127	379	518
Kuwait	..	0.0	100	93	1994	..	3.6	543	..	..
Kyrgyz Republic	10.9	3.2	..	89	1995	..	3.7	12	..	..
Lao PDR	2.5	0.2	..	65	1995	2.6	1.3	5	10	..
Latvia	12.1	2.9	..	85	1994	..	4.4	78	..	..
Lebanon	4.0	1.3	..	88	1992	5.3	2.1	34	87	..
Lesotho	..	0.0	80	82	1994	..	3.5	16	..	..
Liberia	..	..	..	..	..	..	..	..	..	..
Libya	4.1	1.0	100	89	..	..	..	..	..	..
Lithuania	11.9	4.0	..	94	1995	..	5.1	76	..	..
Luxembourg	11.8	2.2	..	80	1993	6.2	6.2	1985	2003	1983
Macao	..	..	..	..	1994	..	..	..	..	..
Macedonia, FYR	5.0	2.1	..	85	1995	8.3	7.3	130	146	..
Madagascar	0.9	0.1	65	59	1995	..	1.1	3	..	..
Malawi	1.6	0.0	80	99	1995	..	2.3	3	..	..
Malaysia	2.0	0.4	88	81	1994	..	1.4	49	..	..

Table A.6 (*continued*)

Country	Health Services Indicators: In-patient beds per 1,000 pop. mr 1990–95	Physicians per 1,000 pop. mr 1990–95	Access to health services, % mr 1990–95	Immunization coverage, measles, % mr 1990–95	Health Finance Indicators: Year	Total health expenditures % of GDP	Health expenditures (public) % of GDP	Health expenditures (public) per cap. US$	Total health expenditures per cap. US$	Total health expenditures PPP$
Maldives	0.8	0.1	..	86	1990	4.9	..	..	..	..
Mali	..	0.1	..	49	1991	2.7	1.2	3	8	15
Malta	5.4	2.5	..	90	..	..	..	..	..	..
Marshall Islands	2.3	..	..	..	..	..	..	..	..	..
Martinique	..	1.7	..	..	..	..	..	..	..	..
Mauritania	0.7	0.1	..	53	1991	5.2	1.1	6	28	75
Mauritius	2.9	..	99	85	1991	3.4	2.1	56	90	408
Mayotte	..	..	..	..	..	..	..	..	..	..
Mexico	0.8	1.3	91	90	1994	5.3	2.8	116	223	365
Micronesia, Fed. Sts.	..	..	..	76	..	..	..	..	..	..
Moldova	12.2	3.5	..	98	1994	..	4.9	16	..	..
Mongolia	11.5	2.7	100	85	1992	4.7	4.4	24	26	174
Montserrat	..	0.5	..	..	1994	5.6	3.1	154	277	..
Morocco	1.1	0.4	62	92	1993	3.4	1.6	17	36	126
Mozambique	0.9	..	30	71	1991	..	4.6	5	..	..
Myanmar	0.6	0.1	..	66	1994	..	0.4	7	..	..
Namibia	5.0	0.2	..	57	1993	7.6	3.9	68	133	303
Nepal	0.2	0.1	..	78	1995	5.0	1.2	2	10	60
Netherlands	11.3	2.5	100	95	1995	8.8	6.8	1495	2258	1825
Netherlands Antilles	..	1.4	..	..	1994	4.8	2.5	194	364	..
New Caledonia	..	..	..	..	..	..	..	..	..	..
New Zealand	7.3	2.1	100	87	1994	7.5	5.7	828	1078	1335
Nicaragua	1.8	0.7	..	81	1994	7.8	4.3	19	34	..
Niger	..	0.0	30	38	1995	..	1.6	4	..	..
Nigeria	1.7	..	67	50	1994	1.4	0.3	1	5	18
Norway	..	3.3	100	93	1994	7.3	6.9	1963	2078	1900
Oman	2.1	0.6	89	98	1991	..	2.5	142	..	..
Pakistan	0.7	0.5	85	53	1991	3.5	0.8	3	13	70
Panama	2.5	1.6	82	84	1994	7.5	5.4	146	201	485
Papua New Guinea	4.0	0.1	96	35	1994	..	2.8	36	..	..
Paraguay	0.6	0.3	..	76	1994	4.3	1.0	17	72	161
Peru	1.4	1.0	..	97	1994	4.9	2.6	56	106	199
Philippines	1.4	0.1	..	86	1991	2.4	1.3	10	17	60
Poland	6.4	2.3	100	96	1992	6.0	5.0	110	134	283
Portugal	4.3	2.9	..	94	1995	8.1	4.5	463	827	1058
Puerto Rico	..	1.8	..	..	..	..	..	..	..	..
Qatar	..	1.5	..	87	1993	2.8	..	..	343	511
Reunion	..	..	..	..	..	..	..	..	..	..
Romania	7.7	1.8	..	93	1994	..	3.6	44	..	..
Russian Federation	11.7	3.8	..	91	1994	4.8	4.1	83	96	225
Rwanda	1.7	..	..	..	1990	..	1.9	7	..	..
Sao Tome & Principe	4.8	0.5	..	69	1995	..	6.2	22	..	..
Saudi Arabia	2.5	1.4	98	94	1991	2.2	..	..	161	202
Senegal	0.7	0.1	40	80	1990	..	1.0	8	..	..
Seychelles	..	..	..	92	1994	..	4.0	272	..	..
Sierra Leone	..	..	..	44	1991	3.6	1.5	3	8	22
Singapore	3.6	1.4	100	88	1994	3.5	1.1	270	621	823
Slovak Republic	7.6	3.0	..	99	1995	..	6.0	196	..	..
Slovenia	5.7	2.1	..	91	1995	..	7.4	555	..	..
Solomon Islands	2.8	0.2	..	76	1991	5.6	3.3	23	39	111
Somalia	0.7	..	..	30	..	..	..	..	..	..
South Africa	..	..	..	76	1993	7.9	3.6	105	233	396
Spain	4.2	4.1	..	90	1995	7.6	6.0	854	1091	1166
Sri Lanka	2.7	..	90	88	1993	1.9	1.4	8	11	61
St. Kitts and Nevis	9.2	0.9	..	100	1994	5.9	3.4	173	298	604
St. Lucia	4.3	0.5	..	94	..	..	..	..	..	..
St. Vincent & the Grenadines	5.0	0.5	..	100	1994	5.9	4.0	86	129	..

Country	Health Services Indicators: *In-patient beds per 1,000 pop. mr 1990–95*	*Physicians per 1,000 pop. mr 1990–95*	*Access to health services, % mr 1990–95*	*Immunization coverage, measles, % mr 1990–95*	Health Finance Indicators: *Year*	*Total health expenditures % of GDP*	*Health expenditures (public) % of GDP*	*Health expenditures (public) per cap. US$*	*Total health expenditures per cap. US$*	*Total health expenditures PPP$*
Sudan	1.1	..	70	74	1991	0.3	..	..	4	..
Suriname	5.7	0.8	..	61	1994	5.0	2.6	1057	2056	259
Swaziland	..	0.1	..	85	1995	..	3.0	35	..	..
Sweden	6.1	3.1	100	96	1994	7.7	6.4	1452	1742	1540
Switzerland	8.7	3.1	100	83	1994	9.6	6.9	2537	3533	2395
Syrian Arab Republic	1.1	0.8	99	98	..	..	..	..	..	..
Taiwan	4.9	1.3	..	..	1993	4.9	2.6	280	522	686
Tajikistan	8.8	2.1	..	90	1994	..	6.4	93	..	..
Tanzania	0.9	..	93	75	1995	..	3.0	4	..	..
Thailand	1.7	0.2	59	87	1992	5.3	1.4	27	103	336
Togo	1.5	0.1	..	65	1991	3.4	1.2	5	15	40
Tonga	..	0.5	..	87	1992	4.0	2.9	42	58	..
Trinidad and Tobago	3.2	0.7	99	87	1994	3.9	2.6	100	151	381
Tunisia	1.8	0.6	90	89	1993	5.9	3.0	51	99	..
Turkey	2.5	1.1	100	75	1994	4.2	2.7	65	99	239
Turkmenistan	10.5	3.2	..	90	1994	..	2.8	62	..	..
Turks & Caicos Isl.	..	0.5	..	..	..	..	..	..	..	..
Uganda	0.9	..	71	79	1994	3.9	1.8	4	10	61
Ukraine	11.8	4.4	100	96	1995	..	5.0	35	..	..
United Arab Emirates	3.1	0.8	90	90	1994	2.5	2.0	307	379	378
United Kingdom	5.1	1.5	..	92	1994	6.9	5.8	1014	1205	1366
United States	4.4	2.5	..	89	1995	14.5	7.0	1614	3828	3873
Uruguay	4.5	3.2	..	80	1994	8.5	2.0	104	439	642
Uzbekistan	8.4	3.3	..	71	1994	..	3.5	5	..	..
Vanuatu	..	0.1	..	66	1993	..	3.3	34	..	..
Venezuela	2.6	1.6	..	94	1994	7.1	2.3	66	202	602
Viet Nam	3.8	0.4	97	95	1993	5.2	1.1	..	..	..
Virgin Islands (UK)	..	1.7	..	..	1994	5.3	2.6	..	862	..
Virgin Islands (US)	4.8	1.7	..	..	..	..	..	..	..	..
West Bank	..	..	..	..	..	..	..	..	..	..
West Bank/Gaza Strip	..	..	..	..	1995	6.2	3.4	63	113	..
Western Samoa	..	..	..	81	1992		3.1	29	..	..
Yemen, Rep.	0.8	0.1	..	49	1994	2.6	1.1	17	39	..
Yugoslavia, Fed. Republic	13.6	4.3	..	75	1994	..	..	..	..	..
Zaire	1.4	0.1	59	41	1990	..	0.2	..	..	..
Zambia	..	0.1	75	78	1990	3.3	2.3	12	17	31
Zimbabwe	0.5	0.1	..	78	1991	6.5	2.3	14	41	122

Note: .. indicates data not available.

ANNEX B

Highlights from Major International Initiatives in HNP

Task Force on Basic Social Services for All

In October 1995, the United Nations Administrative Committee on Coordination (ACC) established the Task Force on Basic Social Services for All to help coordinate the response of the United Nations system to the recommendations of the recent UN conferences and summits. The unifying theme of the system-wide action plan, on which the Task Force is based, is the provision of assistance to countries for a concerted attack on poverty.

The Task Force on Basic Social Services for All (BSSA) is based upon recent United Nations' global conferences and summits, particularly the International Conference on Population and Development (ICPD) in Cairo, 1994; the World Summit for Social Development (WSSD) in Copenhagen, 1995; the Fourth World Conference on Women (FWCW) in Beijing, 1995; and the Second World Conference on Human Settlements (Habitat II) in Istanbul, 1996.[1]

The Task Force is a broad United Nations initiative to galvanize priority goals and objectives emerging from the recent United Nations conferences, and to rationalize and strengthen follow-up mechanisms for delivery of coordinated assistance at the country and regional levels.

The six key areas included for consideration by the Task Force are:

- population, with special emphasis on reproductive health and family planning services;
- primary health care;
- nutrition;
- basic education;
- drinking water and sanitation; and
- shelter

Goals and Selected BSSA Indicators

Percentage of Population with Access to Health Services

All countries should seek to make primary health care, including reproductive health care, available universally by the end of the current decade (ICPD).

1. The members of the Task Force are: the United Nations Population Fund (UNFPA), which serves as Chair; the United Nations Secretariat (Department for Economic and Social Information and Policy Analysis (DESIPA), Department for Policy Coordination and Sustainable Development (DPCSD), and Department of Humanitarian Affairs (DHA); regional commissions (Economic Commission for Africa (ECA), Economic Commission for Europe (ECE), Economic Commission for Latin America and the Caribbean (ECLAC), Economic and Social Commission for Asia and the Pacific (ESCAP) and Economic and Social Commission for Western Asia (ESCWA); Food and Agriculture Organization of the United Nations (FAO); International Labour Organization (ILO); International Monetary Fund (IMF); Office of the United Nations High Commissioner for Refugees (UNHCR); United Nations Centre for Human Settlements (Habitat); United Nations Children's Fund (UNICEF); United Nations Development Fund for Women (UNIFEM); United Nations Development Programme (UNDP); United Nations Educational, Scientific, and Cultural Organization (UNESCO); United Nations Environment Programme (UNEP); United Nations Industrial Development Organization (UNIDO); United Nations International Drug Control Programme (UNDCP); United Nations Relief and Works Agency for Palestine Refugees in the Near East (UNRWA); World Bank; World Food Programme (WFP); and World Health Organization (WHO).

Governments should promote full access to preventive and curative health care to improve the quality of life, especially for vulnerable and disadvantaged groups, in particular women and children (WSSD).

Governments should provide more accessible, available, and affordable primary health-care services of high quality, including sexual and reproductive health care (FWCW).

Family Planning

All countries should seek to provide universal access to a full range of safe and reliable family-planning methods (ICPD).

Underweight Prevalence among Preschool Children

By the year 2000, achieve a reduction of severe and moderate malnutrition among children under five years of age to half of the 1990 level (WSSD and FWCW).

Maternal Mortality Ratio

Countries should strive to effect significant reductions in maternal mortality by 2015: a reduction in maternal mortality by one-half of the 1990 levels by the year 2000 and a further one-half by 2015 (ICPD, WSSD, and FWCW).

Infant Mortality Rate

By the year 2000, reduce mortality rates of infants by one-third of the 1990 level. By 2015, an infant mortality rate below 35 per 1000 births should be achieved (ICPD and WSSD).

Under-5 Mortality Rate

Countries should strive to reduce their under-5 mortality rates by one-third or to 70 per 1,000 live births, whichever is less, by the year 2000. By 2015, all countries should aim to achieve an under-5 mortality rate below 45 per 1,000 (ICPD and WSSD).

Life Expectancy at Birth

By the year 2000, life expectancy of not less than 60 years should be achieved in every country (WSSD).

Countries should aim to achieve by 2005 a life expectancy at birth greater than 70 years and by 2015 a life expectancy at birth greater than 75 years (ICPD).

School Enrollment Ratio

All countries should strive to ensure complete access to primary school or an equivalent level of education for both girls and boys as quickly as possible, and in any case before 2015. Countries that have achieved the goal of universal primary education are urged to extend education and training and facilitate access to and completion of education at secondary school and higher levels (ICPD, WSSD, and FWCW).

Adult Illiteracy Rate

The adult illiteracy rate should be reduced to at least half its 1990 level, with an emphasis on female literacy (WSSD).

Percentage of Population with Access to Safe Water and to Sanitation

Access to safe drinking water in sufficient quantities and proper sanitation for all should be provided (ICPD, WSSD, and Habitat).

Floor Area per Person

The availability of adequate shelter for all should be improved (WSSD and Habitat).

Major International Conferences

In addition to the Task Force on Basic Social Services for All, four international conferences have had a major impact on setting the broad policy agenda for international work in the HNP sector. These include:

- WHO's initiative to achieve *Health For All by the Year 2000 Strategy,* presented at the Thirtieth World Health Assembly in 1977 (enshrined at *Alma Ata*);
- UNICEF's initiative to improve the *State of the World's Children,* presented at the World Summit for Children in 1990;
- UNFPA's initiative to improve *reproductive health,* presented at the International Conference on Population and Development in Cairo in 1994; and
- The World Food Summit in Rome in 1996 and the International Conference on Nutrition in Rome in 1992.

New Direction in Health: Update of the Health For All by the Year 2000 Initiative

The Global Strategy for **Health for All by the Year 2000**, founded on primary health care principles and adopted by the World Health Assembly in 1977, has provided a common health policy framework in the last two decades.

Adopting "health for all" (HFA) as a fundamental objective has committed governments to attain "as a *minimum* by *all* people in *all* countries, *at least* such a level of health that they are capable of working productively and of participating actively in the social life of the community in which they live" (*The World Health Report 1996; Fighting Disease, Fostering Development*).

The **Health for All** goals in countries include:

- at least 5 percent of the gross national product spent on health; a 'reasonable' percentage of the national health expenditure devoted to local health care (reasonable defined by country context);
- equitable distribution of resources, and;
- primary health care available to the whole population.

Primary health care targets by year 2000 include:

- access to safe water (85 percent);
- adequate sanitary facilities in the home (75 percent);
- immunization (90 percent);
- local health care (first-level facilities) with at least 20 essential drugs (85 percent); and
- trained personnel for pregnancy, childbirth, and caring for children up to at least one year of age (100 percent).

In addition to disease-specific mortality and morbidity targets, specified goals for the year 2000 are:

- Infant mortality rate less than 50 per 1,000 live births;
- Probability of dying before fifth birthday less than 70 per 1000 live births; and
- Maternal mortality (per 100,000 live births) to be reduced to 50 percent of 1990 level.

To assess the global progress in the attainment of HFA at the end of the decade, and to set a new direction in health, WHO is currently evaluating the original global targets (economic, demographic, social, nutritional, lifestyle, water supply and sanitation, human and financial resources, drugs, maternal and child health, family planning, life expectancy, mortality, morbidity, and disability). The evaluation will contribute to a revised HFA policy for action beyond 2000.

New Directions in Caring for the World's Children: The 1990 World Summit for Children

The 1990 *World Summit for Children* set goals for reducing deaths, malnutrition, disease, and disability among the children of the developing world.

The end-of-century goals, agreed to by almost all the world's governments following the Summit, can be summarized by ten priority points:

- A one-third reduction in 1990 under-5 death rates (or 70 per 1,000 live births, whichever is less).
- A halving of 1990 maternal mortality rates.
- A halving of 1990 rates of malnutrition among the world's under-5s (to include the elimination of micronutrient deficiencies, support for breastfeeding by all maternity units, and a reduction in the incidence of low birth weight to less than 10 percent).
- The achievement of 90 percent immunization among children under the age of one, the eradication of polio, the elimination of neonatal tetanus, a 90 percent reduction in measles cases, and a 95 percent reduction in measles deaths (compared to pre-immunization levels).
- A halving of child deaths caused by diarrheal disease.
- A one-third reduction in child deaths from acute respiratory infections.
- Basic education for all children and completion of primary education by at least 80 percent—girls as well as boys.
- Clean water and safe sanitation for all communities.
- Acceptance in all countries of the Convention on the Rights of the Child, including improved protection for children in especially difficult circumstances.
- Universal access to high quality family planning information and services in order to prevent pregnancies that are too early, too closely spaced, too late, or too numerous.

UNICEF has one of the most detailed programs for monitoring and tracking progress of any of the international organizations. The latest annual report—the *State of the World's Children 1996*—provides some striking illustrations of both successes and failures during this decade in achieving these goals. A major achievement has been improvements in securing access to safe water for rural populations:

Safe Water Access	1980	1990
Sub-Saharan Africa	22%	38%
North Africa and Middle East	30%	51%
Latin America	42%	52%
South East Asia	41%	53%
South Asia	31%	66%

New Directions in Population and Reproductive Health: The 1994 International Conference on Population and Development in Cairo

The 1994 *International Conference on Population and Development* (ICPD) in Cairo, has set the agenda for addressing population issues as we enter the 21st century. Several key changes in population dynamics and in the policy environment have led to an international consensus on the approach to population and reproductive health.

Major development objectives expressed at the Conference are to:

- ***Bridge*** the gender gap in education;
- ***Promote*** equity for women;
- ***Reduce*** maternal mortality and morbidity;
- ***Increase*** child survival; and
- ***Provide*** universal access to reproductive health and family planning services.

The ICPD approach does not abandon population issues but puts individual needs first by:

- continuing to assist the world's poorest countries as they complete the demographic transition (slowing population growth) during the next few years (high birth rates and very young populations make it more difficult to reduce poverty and pursue sustainable economic development);
- integrating population policies more effectively with core development agendas such as seeking better infant and child health, educating girls and empowering women (understanding the social, economic, and political dimensions of urbanization, international migration, and aging);
- providing the poor with access to high quality and user-oriented (culturally sensitive) services that offer a range of choices in addressing population and reproductive health needs; and
- redefining the role of the state in population policies (selective investments in service delivery infrastructure and institution building in very poor countries), while limiting activities to providing information and improving the functioning of the private sector in more advanced middle-income countries.

The Bank's role in the implementation of the recommendations from this conference is described in greater details in the Bank publication *Population and Development: Implications for the World Bank*, 1994.

New Directions in Nutrition: The 1996 World Food Summit

The 1996 *World Food Summit* in Rome—and its nutritional antecedents the World Summit for Children and the 1992 International Conference on Nutrition in Rome—came to a consensus on the causality of malnutrition: **food, disease, and behavior**.

The World Food Summit emphasized the intersectoral nature of effective nutrition policies. Unlike other health problems, including maternal and reproductive health, problems in malnutrition are not well addressed through health services alone. Instead major reforms to address malnutrition need to focus on policies in five major intersectoral areas:

- ***Policy and institutional framework*** to support agricultural and rural development;
- ***New role of the state,*** with an emphasis away from heavy public intervention in the rural economy, towards providing the enabling, sound macro-economic, fiscal, and sectoral policy environments;
- ***Private sector involvement*** to mobilize the needed investment capital, production, and services;
- ***Community and local government participation*** in designing and implementing nutrition policies rather than relying on the central government; and
- ***Partnerships*** at all levels of involvement, ranging from central governments to local governments to community participation to the private sector.

The World Summit for Children set specific quantitative goals for the year 2000 for nutrition, which remain in force today. The International Conference on Nutrition broadened the anti-hunger strategy to include food production, poverty alleviation, and nutrition-friendly trade policies, in addition to the targeted nutrition interventions highlighted at the World Food Summit.

Countries implementing prioritized and budgeted nutrition policies include China, Indonesia, Tanzania, and Zimbabwe. Promising new policy formulation and implementation is taking place in a broad range of countries including Albania, Bolivia, Burkina Faso, Mexico, Peru, South Africa, Sri Lanka, Zambia, and Bangladesh.

Much remains to be done. The next generation of nutrition action plans will include comprehensive food policy reforms, heavy investment in communications for behavioral change in nutrition, greater involvement of private food industry, and reduced reliance on untargeted, stand-alone food distribution programs.

ANNEX C

Essential Health, Nutrition, and Population Services

Essential HNP Services

The old enemies of the poor include malnutrition, high fertility, communicable diseases, childhood illnesses, and maternal and perinatal conditions. More than half of the disease burden in Sub-Saharan Africa and South Asia can be addressed effectively through local adaptation of interventions such as immunization, integrated management of childhood illness, family planning, maternal and perinatal health care, food fortification, targeted nutrition programs, and school health.

As populations age, the disease burden and cost of treating non-communicable conditions and injuries becomes increasingly important. Ensuring universal access to a limited range of public and private services that address these conditions, and that are affordable in low-income countries, helps not only the poor but also helps others avoid impoverishment due to illness (see Figure C.1 adapted from Bulletin of WHO 1995, 73:735–740).

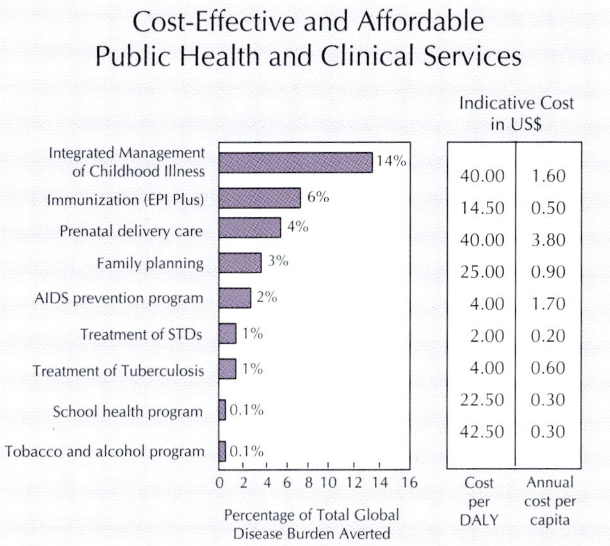

FIGURE C.1

Immunization Policies

Three of the world's poorest countries—Bangladesh, India, and Viet Nam—have improved immunization coverage by over 25 percent since 1988 through effective vaccination programs. Preventing childhood diseases through such programs remains one of the best investments that countries can make to improve health for the poor. The cost is generally just US$12-30 per disability-adjusted life year (DALY).

Although immunization saves about 9 million lives a year worldwide, 2 million children still die from current immunization-preventable diseases. Furthermore, UNICEF estimates that a total of 16 million people of all age groups could be saved if currently available vaccines were deployed effectively against all vaccine-preventable infectious diseases. Most of the effective vaccines currently in use have been available for the past 15 years. Yet, due to poor policies and problems in implementation, immunization coverage is leveling off

The 200th Anniversary of Vaccine Discovery

On the 200th anniversary of the discovery of vaccines by the English physician Edward Jenner in 1796, 44 low- and middle-income countries had already reached the year 2000 target of 90 percent coverage set by UNICEF.

The successful eradication of smallpox saves 5 million lives annually. Other infectious illnesses such as measles (which currently kills 1.1 million children a year) could also be eliminated or at least controlled at low levels with proper policies.

The year 2000 has been set as the target date by WHO and UNICEF for the eradication of polio. Polio no longer occurs in the Americas, China, and many other countries.

The policy challenge for low- and middle-income countries is to institutionalize immunizations within each country's health program and develop national self-sufficiency in running these programs as part of essential and affordable health services.

Can low-income countries afford to pay for such vaccination programs?

The answer is yes!

Already, 20 low- and middle-income countries pay their own vaccine bills. They include large and poor countries such as China, Egypt, and Indonesia. A further 15 nations pay over half of their own vaccine costs.

in many countries and falling in others, with the global rates having peaked at less than 80 percent according to UNICEF estimates.

Integrated Management of Childhood Illnesses

When children get sick they often have more than one illness. By using treatment protocols that integrate the management of all the major causes of childhood illness and death (diarrhea, pneumonia, malnutrition, measles, and malaria), misdiagnosis and incorrect treatment are reduced. Such protocols can be taught through a single course that facilitates the development of an integrated approach to child health rather than a diagnosis-specific programmatic approach.

Integrated management of childhood illnesses combines prevention (feeding advice, immunization, and vitamin A) with cure. It uses a short list of effective and affordable essential drugs, making life-saving treatment accessible to the poor. It helps doctors, nurses, and other health care providers to make more accurate diagnoses and to know when to refer difficult cases. And it emphasizes the need for better communications skills when dealing with sick children and their mothers. This approach is now being successfully introduced in Bolivia, Ethiopia, Indonesia, Nepal, Peru, Philippines, Tanzania, Uganda, and Zambia. Many other countries have taken the first steps towards adopting this approach.

Reproductive Health

Each year, more than 200 million women become pregnant. Of these more than 50 million experience acute pregnancy-related complications, 15 million develop long-term disabilities, and 585,000 die (see Figure C.2, adapted from UNICEF 1996).

Deaths in Pregnancy and Childbirth

Daily Toll

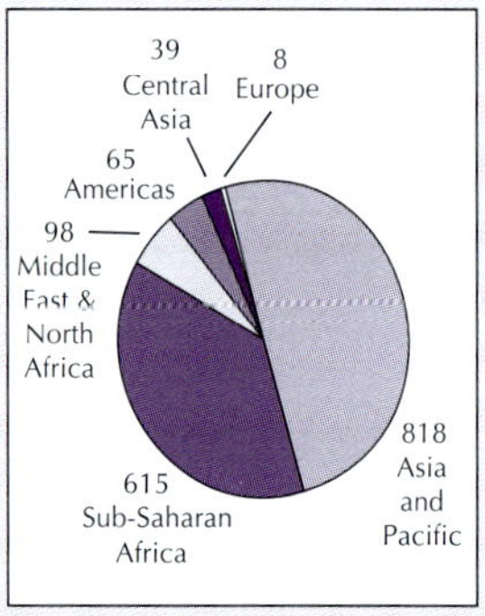

	Maternal deaths per year
Europe	3,000
Central Asia	14,000
Americas	23,000
M. East & N. Africa	35,000
Sub-Saharan Africa	219,000
Asia and Pacific	291,000
WORLD	585,000

FIGURE C.2

In addition, poor maternal health and nutritional status, and inappropriate management of labor and delivery, are responsible for 75 percent of the 7.5 million annual perinatal deaths. This continues to be one of the most neglected health problems in the world for which effective and affordable interventions have been available for decades. What is lacking are appropriate policies to help families know when to seek health care and to ensure that they have access to quality obstetric care when needed.

Additional policies on reproductive health have evolved out of the recommendations of the 1994 International Conference on Population and Development in Cairo. These include:

- linking reproductive health policies to girls' education, the status of women, and overall poverty reduction (e.g. Pakistan and Sri Lanka);
- preventing unwanted pregnancies through information and contraceptive choice, and by training female workers at the community level in providing family planning (e.g. Tunisia and Bangladesh);
- facilitating safe pregnancy, deliveries, and motherhood by preventing and managing pregnancy complications and by eliminating unsafe abortions (e.g. Romania);
- promoting positive health practices such as safe sex, early treatment of sexually transmitted diseases, delayed marriages, birth spacing, and education (e.g. Senegal);
- preventing harmful practices such as genital mutilation, discrimination, and domestic violence (e.g. Ghana).

Nutrition

Three types of nutrition problems predominate in low- and middle-income countries:

- *Undernutrition*—Overall inadequacy of food intake to meet needs for growth, immune function, cognitive development, and reproduction affects 30 percent of children and 25 percent of women, while 56 percent of all under-5 deaths is indirectly associated with some form of malnutrition (see Figure C.3, adapted from WHO Division for Child Health Development);
- *Micronutrient Malnutrition*—Insufficiency of essential vitamins (e.g. Vitamins A, D, and folic acid) and minerals (e.g. iron and iodine) in the diet affects 1 billion people worldwide;
- *Overnutrition*—Excess intake of calories relative to energy requirements and an imbalanced intake of other nutrients (generally excess fat and insufficient fiber) are still small but growing problems, particularly in middle-income countries and poor urban areas.

Deaths in Children Under 5
in Low- and Middle-Income Countries

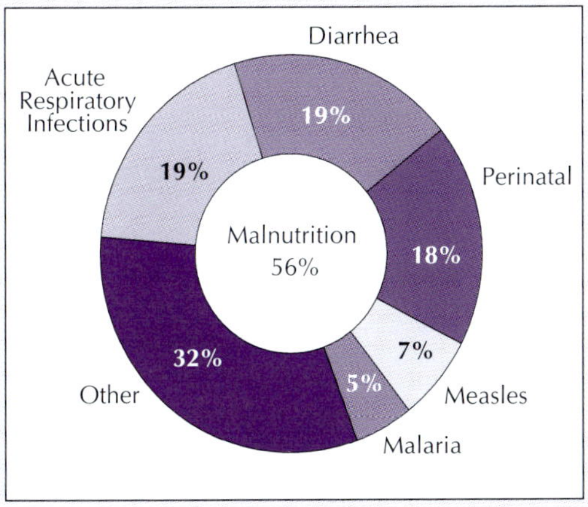

FIGURE C.3

Malnutrition is the result of an interaction between food intake, disease risk factors, and behavior.

The quality and quantity of food is a function of household purchasing power (including subsistence production), food prices, and food preferences and beliefs. Disease is the product of both exposure to disease, resistance, and treatment (including dietary management) at home, and medical interventions. Frequent diseases associated with anorexia, fever, and diarrhea have the greatest effect on nutrition. Malnutrition, in turn, reduces resistance to disease. Nutritional behaviors—including breastfeeding, active feeding of toddlers, energy expenditure, avoidance of empty calories, and frequency of meals for youngsters—determine how well an individual is nourished at any given income level and for any given disease environment.

The policy and programmatic options for dealing with malnutrition must address these constraints. Increasing the family's food purchasing power is critical where food insecurity is a major determinant of malnutrition. This can be done through increasing employment, microcredit and microenterprise, improving the efficiency of food production and marketing, encouraging food industry development, or through targeted interventions and social transfer programs. But increasing income alone is not enough to improve nutrition within a generation—nutrition education to change behavior is needed to accelerate the impact of income on nutrition.

Reducing the effect of disease on nutrition involves immunization, improved water supply and sanitation, improved hygiene, and access to minimum nutrition inputs in the context of health care (growth promotion, nutritional care of the sick child, micronutrient supplements, breastfeeding promotion, dietary advice, and care of the acutely malnourished child). Addressing malnutrition also requires changing behaviors of policymakers, bureaucrats, service providers, community leaders, and beneficiaries, through individual counseling, information dissemination, social marketing, taxation/subsidies, regulation, advertising, and public relations.

Interventions to deal with nutrition problems require action at both the macroeconomic and community level, involving many sectors beyond the purview of health or agriculture. Some of the most successful interventions include:

- community-level programs with heavy emphasis on behavioral change and linked to other sectors as needed (education, agriculture, health, and childcare in Indonesia, Tamil Nadu, Tanzania, Thailand, and Zimbabwe);
- targeted income transfer or food marketing programs that enable the poor to obtain more food (Brazil, Colombia, Honduras); and
- micronutrient programs (salt iodization in Ecuador, vitamin A supplementation in Indonesia, iron fortification of flour in Venezuela).

School Health and Nutrition

There are more children at school today than ever before in human history, due to the success of child survival strategies and global efforts to achieve universal basic education. The accessibility of this school-age population contributes to the cost-effectiveness of some school-based health, nutrition, and reproductive programs. Simple preventive services (health education, family planning, and micronutrient supplementation) and curative services (deworming, first aid) can improve health for an age class that is often underserved by the health systems of the poor, and will allow children to take fuller advantage of what is often their only opportunity for formal education. Participatory health education for schoolchildren (counseling on targeted tobacco use, violence, and reproductive health) is one of the most timely and effective ways of promoting healthier life styles, and of averting the emerging pandemic of non-communicable disease among the next generation of poor.

Successful school health programs (e.g. Dominican Republic and Guinea) require intersectoral partnerships, and depend on the existing educational infrastructure for aspects of service delivery. The health sector remains responsible for technical oversight, including program design, training, monitoring at the community level, and supporting referral systems.

Re-emerging or New Communicable Diseases

Increasing human mobility and the spread of antimicrobial resistance have contributed to increased threats from tuberculosis, malaria, and HIV/AIDS infections—without respect for national borders (e.g. Sub-Saharan Africa). Prevention and treatment policies must be adapted to keep up with these trends.

In tuberculosis control, the Directly-Observed Treatment, Short-course (DOTS) strategy has been highly effective in detecting and curing patients, and preventing drug resistance (e.g., China, India, Peru, and Tanzania). Malaria control now relies on a combination of approaches, such as treatment combined with insecticide-treated mosquito nets, and less on household spraying. Such bed-nets have been shown to reduce under-5 mortality by 20 percent in several Sub-Saharan African countries (e.g. Gambia).

Finally, new approaches in the control and treatment of sexually transmitted diseases have already contributed to controlling the incidence of the HIV/AIDS pandemic (e.g. Tanzania, Thailand, and Uganda).

Non-Communicable Diseases

In the near future, non-communicable diseases (NCDs)—led mainly by cardiovascular diseases, cancers, and mental illness—and injuries will add to the list of common afflictions that burden the poor and that escalate costs of health care systems.

Tobacco is the most prominent cause of NCDs, along with alcohol abuse and intake of foods high in saturated fat. In many middle-income countries, cardiovascular diseases are already the leading cause of death, and in low-income countries they are becoming increasingly important. Tobacco is a particularly difficult development challenge because:

- annual deaths from tobacco will increase significantly over the next three decades, exceeding combined deaths from AIDS, tuberculosis, and the complications of childbirth by 2025 (see Figure C.4 adapted from Global Burden of Disease);
- half of tobacco deaths will occur during people's productive lives (35-69), with an average loss of 20 to 25 years of life;
- tobacco consumption is most common among the poor, rising rapidly in low-income countries;
- related diseases are expensive to treat and they compete for funding with other priority areas; and
- tobacco causes at least a US$200 billion net economic loss globally, or about 1 percent of world GDP.

The prevalence of debilitating or fatal injuries—due to road accidents, gender-based violence, homicide, and

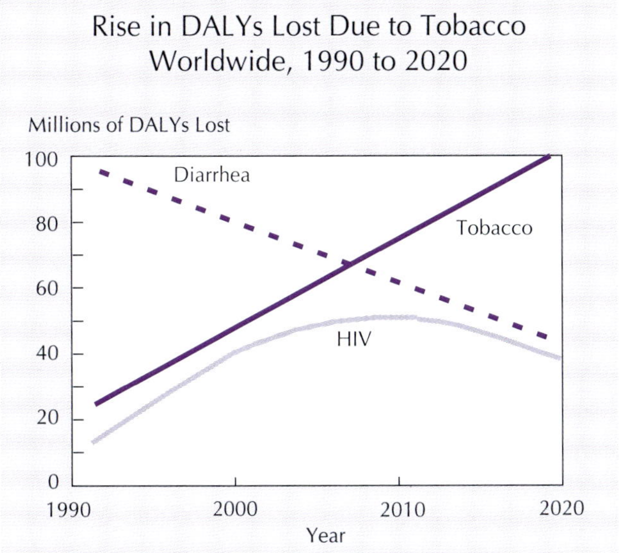

FIGURE C.4

suicide—will continue to rise. Current experience shows that alcohol and other intoxicants are major contributing factors. Road injuries could become the third biggest cause of disability and death by the year 2020 (comprising 5 percent of the burden of disease). Often it is the world's poor who are most adversely affected by these conditions since they have less access to quality curative health services.

The best responses to NCDs and injuries are largely policy-based. These include:

- Encouraging tobacco control with: (a) high prices; (b) serious and prominent health warnings, as in Thailand; (c) complete bans on advertising and promotion of all tobacco-associated products or trademarks, as done in Turkey and Slovenia; (d) focused mass media education messages; (e) increasing capacity to monitor tobacco burdens and control responses and to lobby for control; (f) restrictions on the ability of the tobacco industry to target young smokers and the poor.
- Providing low-cost clinical treatments for those with existing clinical conditions. For example, aspirin, beta-blockers, and diuretics cost about US$1 to US$5 per month, and reduce mortality after a major cardiovascular event by about 25 percent.
- Not subsidizing meat or saturated fat production in countries with prevalent heart disease, because such subsidies may help the rich more than the poor, and because of adverse health impacts in these populations. Mortality from coronary heart disease fell by more than one-third among Polish men and women from 1991 to 1993, largely because of declines in intake of saturated fat. These dietary changes occurred when the government ended subsidies for meat and dairy products, chiefly butter subsidies.
- Inter-sectoral coordination, legislation, and mass education for road safety.
- Undertaking appropriate research and development for these NCDs and injuries, including improved epidemiological and economic studies, and better low-cost treatment and management algorithms.

Core Population-Based Preventive Services

Central to the management of all population health priorities is an infrastructure that sustains specific technical capability in health promotion and disease control. Such an infrastructure includes primary and continuing professional education in population-based health skills such as epidemiology, biostatistics, policy analysis and development, media communications, health education, environmental and occupational health, and cultural awareness (see Figure C.5 for the process of affecting communication change).

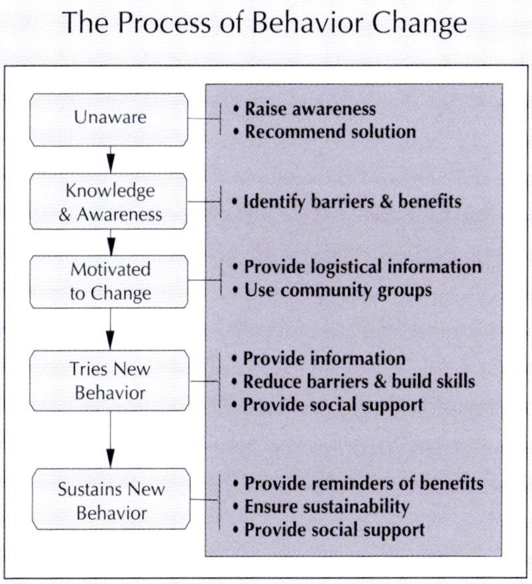

FIGURE C.5

An educated health workforce can best apply the core functions of population health delivery. These core functions include (a) assessment: the identification, quantification, and description of population health problems;

(b) policy development: regulation, analysis, advocacy, and political action; and (c) assurance: evaluation and improvement of policies and interventions intended to solve health problems. Thus, population approaches may support direct individual service delivery to ensure that all persons identified as at risk for a given health problem have access to and utilize an intervention. More importantly, the population health infrastructure is responsible for leadership, policy development, and analytic work necessary to solve problems that impact on the larger public good.

Finally, it must be emphasized that the nature of the population health approach is inherently political. For example, the poor are adversely affected by market forces that seek to sell harmful products, and thus, political action is necessary to contain these forces, just as environmental action is necessary to contain vectors of communicable diseases such as mosquitoes.

Communication and information dissemination mobilize public opinion to support not only changes in personal health behavior but changes in population-based health matters. Regulation, taxation, and targeted interventions often evolve from political action at the community and national level. Thus, intersectoral collaboration must include a political effort, driven ultimately by a trained population health infrastructure that identifies population health problems.

Several of these population health problems are particularly amenable to behavior change, policy, and other public health approaches. They have been identified as preventable risk factors by Murray and Lopez in *The Global Burden of Disease*, 1996 (see Figure C.6). These risk factors accounted for almost 20 million preventable deaths and for almost 40 percent of DALYs in 1990. Many governments are trying to incorporate this set of risk factors in their country-specific health program strategies.

Global Burden of Disease and Injury Attributable to Selected Risk Factors

Risk Factor	Deaths (mil)	% of total deaths	YLLs (mil)	% of total YLLs	YLDs (mil)	% of total YLDs	DALYs (mil)	% of total DALYs
Malnutrition	5	11.7	199	22.0	200	4.2	219	15.9
Poor water, Sanitation	3	5.3	85	9.4	8	1.7	93	6.8
Unsafe sex	1	2.2	28	3.0	21	4.5	49	3.5
Tobacco	3	6.0	26	2.9	10	2.1	36	2.6
Alcohol	1	1.5	20	2.1	28	6.0	48	3.5
Occupation	1	2.2	22	2.5	15	3.3	38	2.7
Hypertension	3	5.8	18	1.9	1	0.3	20	1.4
Inactivity	2	3.9	11	1.3	2	0.5	14	1.0
Illicit drugs	.1	0.2	3	0.3	6	1.2	8	0.6
Air pollution	.5	1.1	6	0.6	2	0.3	7	0.5

YLD = Years of Life Disabled
YLL = Years of Life Lost
DALY = Disability-Adjusted Life Year

FIGURE C.6

ANNEX D

World Bank Organizational Charts

The World Bank Group

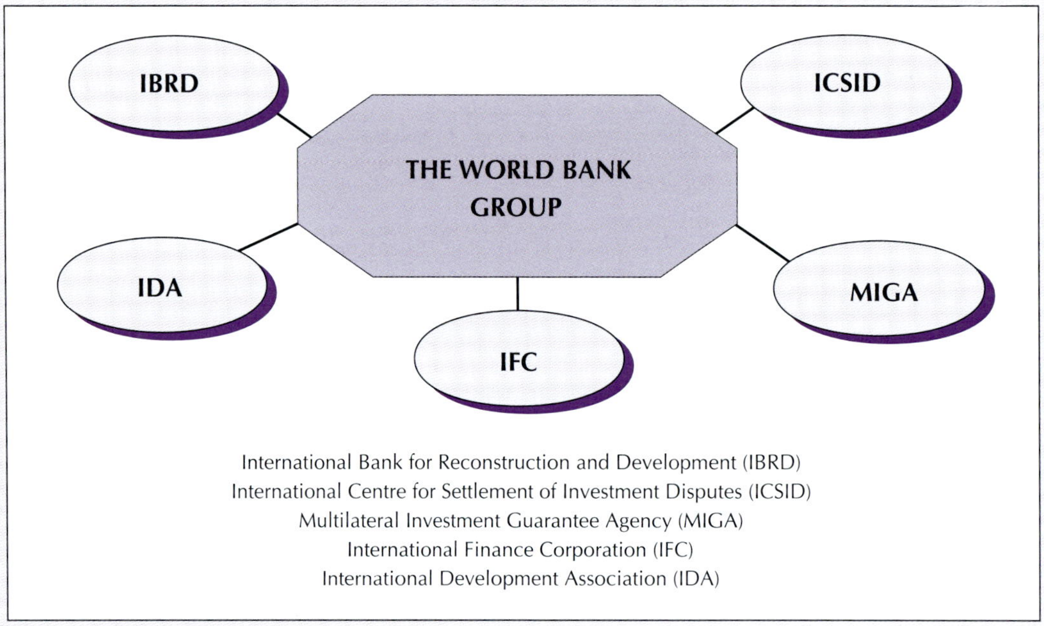

FIGURE D.1

Bank Senior Management and New Technical Networks

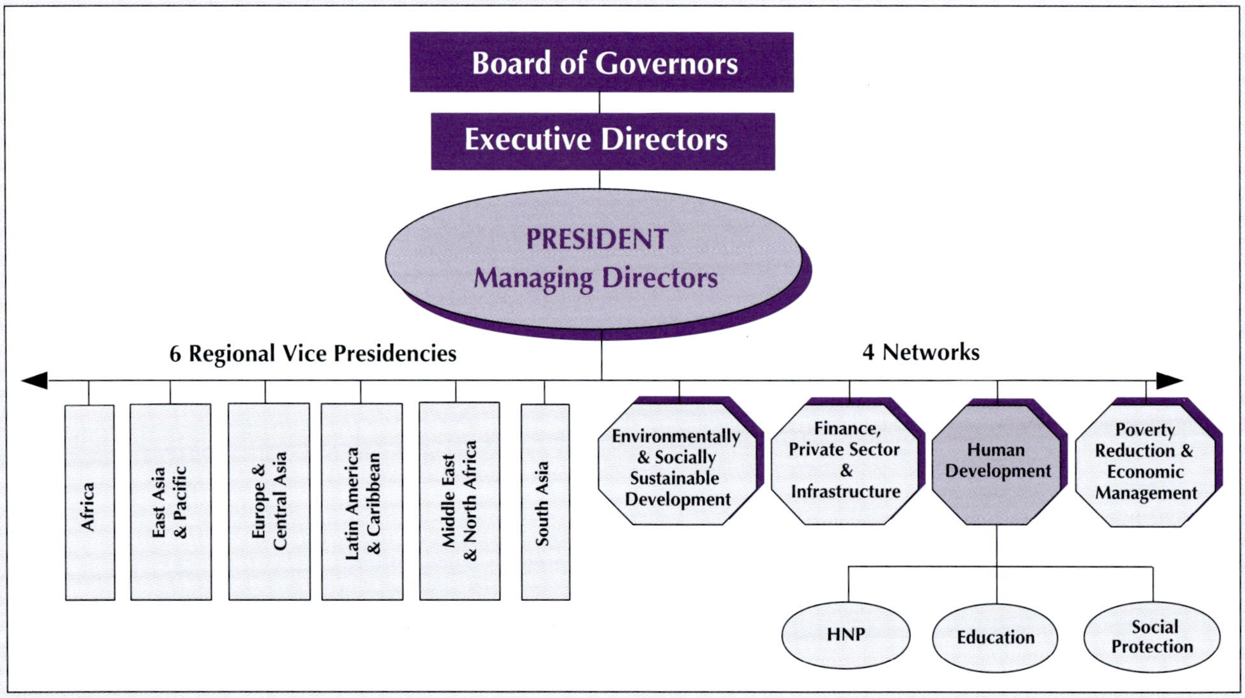

FIGURE D.2

ANNEX E

HNP Sector Portfolio and Management Indicators

Introduction

This Annex presents a set of selected indicators for Bank portfolio performance and management based on the standard CAS presentation, adapted for the purpose of this cross-cutting Sector Strategy Paper. A brief discussion and statistical data are provided under each of the following categories:

- IBRD/IDA Lending to HNP and Other Sectors
- Status of IBRD/IDA Operations in HNP
- IFC and MIGA Operations in HNP
- Country-Specific Analytical Work in HNP
- Selected Portfolio Performance Indicators

HD Lending Reaches 24 Percent of Total Bank Lending in FY96

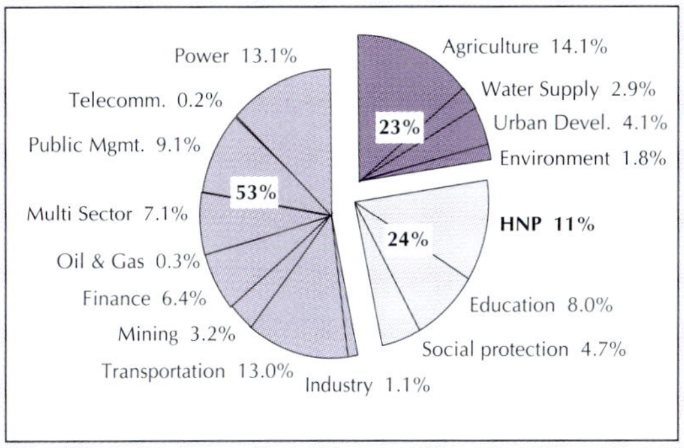

FIGURE E.1

IBRD/IDA Lending to HNP and Other Sectors

This section compares HNP lending to overall Bank lending. During the past ten years alone, annual lending directed towards sectors that have a major impact on health, nutrition, and reproductive outcomes (HNP, education, social protection) increased from about US$1 billion in 1986 to over US$5 billion in FY96, or from 8 to 24 percent of the US$21 billion in new loans (see Figure E.1 and Table E.1).

During the past ten years, cumulative HNP lending has tripled compared with Bank lending to other sectors, increasing from less than 1 percent of total cumulative lending in FY86 to more than 3 percent in FY96 (see Figure E.2). Annual lending to the HNP sector in FY96 reached a record high of 11 percent of Bank lending or US$2.4 billion in new commitments (see discussion below for more details).

In addition to activities that have a direct impact on health, nutrition, and population outcomes, an additional 23 percent of total Bank lending is devoted to agriculture, water supply, environment, and rural/urban development, all of which have an indirect impact on HNP outcomes.

Status of IBRD/IDA Operations in HNP

This section provides information on the sectoral distribution of the Bank's current lending and proposed

Cumulative HNP Portfolio As Share of Overall Bank Lending

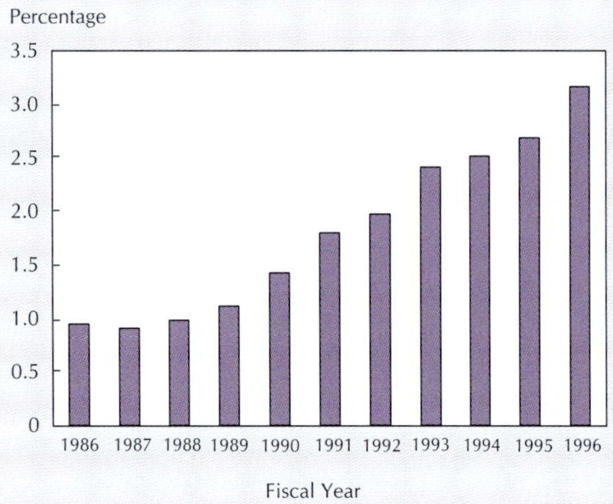

FIGURE E.2

FY86 to FY97: New Commitments and Disbursements in HNP Sector

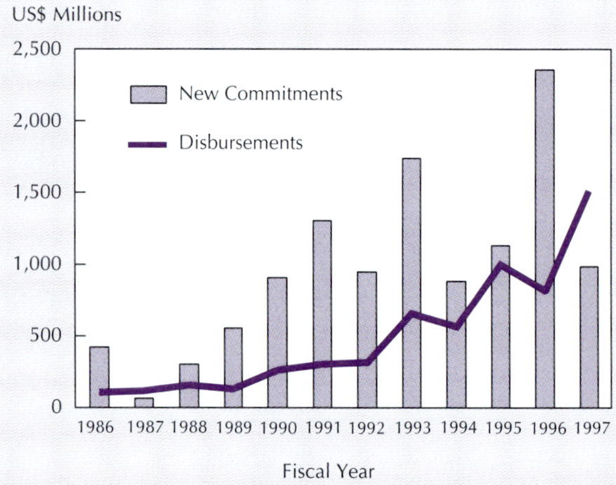

FIGURE E.3

pipeline in the HNP sector (see Table E.2). The Bank's activities in the HNP sector have grown steadily during the past decade to the point where it is now the single largest external financier in low- to middle-income countries, with 154 active projects in 82 countries and an active portfolio value of US$9.2 billion at the end of FY96 (1996 prices). About 48 percent of Bank financing from FY94 to FY96 in HNP was in the form of IDA credits, targeted to poor countries.

Although the cumulative portfolio value has continued to rise, it varies considerably from year to year. FY96 was a record high, with US$2.4 billion in new commitments (see Figure E.3). The reason for the marked increase in FY96 was the approval of five unusually large loans (ranging from US$270 to US$350 million and above) in Argentina, Brazil, India, Mexico, and Russia, bringing the average loan size to US$102 million compared with the usual US$50 to US$60 million range for the sector.

FY97 approvals for HNP are expected to be around US$0.9 billion. This decrease in new commitments compared with FY96 reflects several factors: (a) a return to 16 new projects per year, similar to the FY94 levels (all regions except SAS were affected, but the drop was most pronounced in LAC and MNA); (b) intensified supervision efforts during FY97 in response to recommendations by the Quality Assurance Group that the Bank carry out a portfolio cleanup during FY97; and (c) reallocation of staff resources to set up the new professional networks.

There are good reasons to believe that past growth in the HNP sector will continue and that the consolidation that took place in FY97 is a temporary phenomenon. Based on the planned pipeline, there will be strong continued growth during FY98–FY00, with an expected annual lending of about US$1.5 billion and approximately 22 new projects per year. As of June 97, cumulative disbursements in the HNP sector amounted to US$5.4 billion and the total undisbursed amount was US$6.2 billion. Disbursements in HNP for FY97 are expected to reach US$1.5 billion. A major challenge for the HNP sector is to sustain the anticipated growth without compromising quality and development impact.

The population size of member countries varies from less than 1 million (e.g. Virgin Islands) to more than 1 billion (e.g. China). Both the Bank's budget resources and lending commitments per capita have in the past favored smaller countries (see Figure E.4). Since over 90 percent of the world's poor live in twelve of the Bank's largest client countries, this lending pattern must be adjusted to target poverty groups more effectively in the future.

There are also significant regional variations in past total lending and the future pipeline. The South Asia and LAC regions are major users of HNP lending, current and projected (see Figure E.5). South Asia has 13 completed projects, 23 that are active, and seven in the pipeline for approval in FY98 through FY99. Many of the countries in the ECA region only joined the Bank

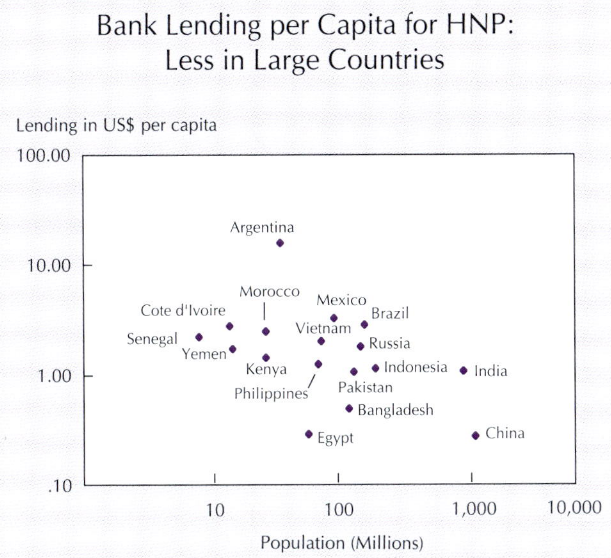

FIGURE E.4

during the past five to ten years. This has led to a rapid rise in commitments in that region. Lending to East Asia could fall during the next three years, as some countries become ineligible for IDA credits and must consider IBRD loan terms.

IFC and MIGA Operations in HNP

IFC approvals in the health sector declined from US$61 million in FY94 to US$30 million in FY95 and to US$1 million in FY96 (See Table E.3). However, it is anticipated that IFC activity in the health sector will increase in the near future. MIGA does not have an HNP Program.

Country-Specific Analytical Work in HNP

This section provides information on country-specific analytical work (see Table E.4). A total of US$3.9 million was spent on country-specific analytical studies or economic and sector work (ESW) in FY96, about 5 percent of spending on ESW Bank-wide.

Selected Portfolio Performance Indicators

This section provides information on selected HNP portfolio performance indicators (see Table E.5). As described in Chapter II, the current HNP lending portfolio is keeping pace with Bank-wide averages in terms of the number of projects rated successful in terms of development objectives and implementation progress (see Figure E.6).

HNP loans grew in size from an average of US$21 million per loan in FY81 to about US$102 million in FY96, both amounts expressed in 1996 prices. The FY96 Bank average per project was US$83 million. FY96 was, however, an unusual year in this respect. In FY97, the average loan size in the HNP sector was about US$60 million. This is still up from the US$45 million loan average in FY95. Resources allocated to the preparation

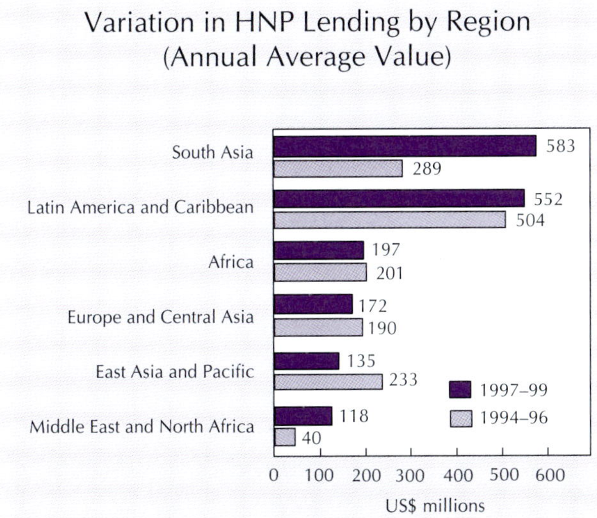

FIGURE E.5

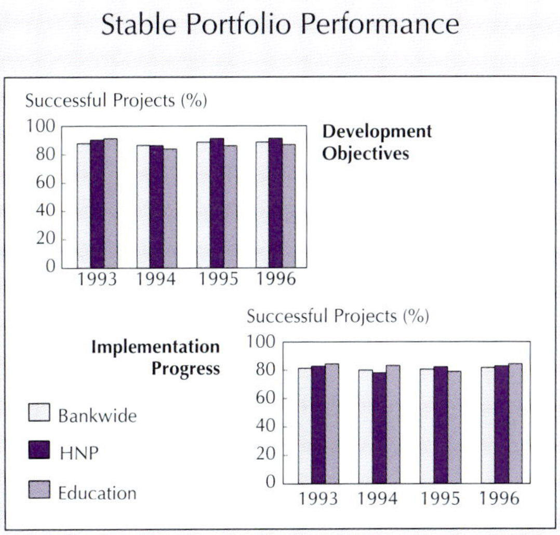

FIGURE E.6

and supervision of HNP operations has grown, but less rapidly than the average loan size (see Table E.5).

A further test of the performance of the portfolio is the ability of the Bank to mobilize additional resources for the HNP sector through domestic and other donor resources. There are some notable success stories in this respect. For example, the Bangladesh Fourth Population Project (FY92) includes IDA financing of US$180 million, complemented by US$165 million from the government and US$256 million from a consortium of 11 donor organizations. Thus the project mobilizes 3.3 times as much resources as the IDA credit. Another example is the Zimbabwe Second Family Health Project. In this case, the IBRD financing of US$25 million was matched by US$53 million from the government and US$37 million from a consortia of five donors.

These efficiency measures are affected by the use of consultant trust funds as a major source of support for HNP project preparation. Trust funds allow managers to free up Bank resources for sector work and project supervision. Today, such trust funds add over a third to the Bank's own administrative budget in the HNP sector (see Figure E.7).

The HNP sector has also been more successful than the Bank on average in mobilizing external budgetary resources, especially Japanese Trust Funds. In the Africa region, for example, trust funds that support HNP work exceeded the available Bank administrative budget in FY97.

Increased Reliance on Trust Funds for Core Administrative Functions

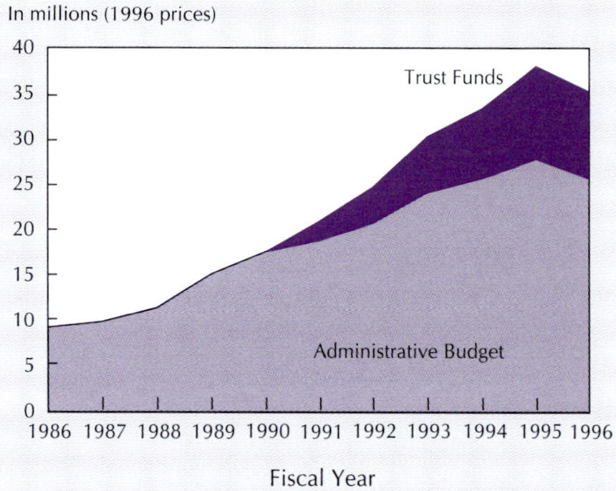

FIGURE E.7

Table E.1 IBRD/IDA Lending Program, FY 1994–2000

	Past			Current	Planned[a]		
Category	FY94	FY95	FY96	FY97	FY98	FY99	FY00
Commitments (US$m)	20,836.0	22,521.7	21,352.2	19,559.5	28,086.7	33,128.6	26,940.9
Sector (%)[b]							
Agriculture	17.0	9.3	11.8	18.5	13.0	14.8	13.0
Education	10.4	9.3	8.0	5.2	8.6	8.7	7.1
Electric Power & Energy	7.7	10.0	13.1	9.8	10.9	10.1	8.2
Environment	4.9	3.7	4.1	1.1	2.3	5.9	6.3
Finance	7.2	13.6	6.7	6.2	6.0	6.4	3.7
Industry	3.1	1.3	1.2	1.0	0.6	2.7	0.4
Mining	0.1	0.1	3.2	1.6	3.7	0.0	0.0
Multisector	6.9	13.8	7.0	11.0	9.1	5.7	2.6
Oil & Gas	5.5	2.7	0.3	0.7	2.9	0.3	3.0
Population, Health, Nutrition	4.3	5.0	11.0	5.1	4.5	8.9	11.3
Public Sector Management	3.4	3.9	8.8	6.1	6.3	4.5	5.7
Social Sector	0.9	4.1	4.7	7.0	4.2	3.1	4.8
Telecommunications	2.0	1.4	0.2	0.0	0.4	0.1	0.0
Transportation	15.9	9.8	13.0	19.1	14.5	15.0	18.4
Urban Development	6.0	7.7	4.1	4.2	6.6	6.8	7.4
Water Supply & Sanitation	4.7	4.4	2.9	3.5	6.5	6.9	8.0
TOTAL	100.0	100.0	100.0	100.0	100.0	100.0	100.0
Lending instrument (%)							
Adjustment loans[c]	13.8	23.6	21.1	26.0	16.9	10.9	7.9
Specific investment loans and others	86.2	76.4	78.9	74.0	83.1	89.1	92.1
TOTAL	100.0	100.0	100.0	100.0	100.0	100.0	100.0
Disbursements (US$m)							
Adjustment loans[c]	4303.7	4710.5	4726.9	4228.4	800.4	111.1	12.0
Specific investment loans and others	11687.4	13665.8	14043.8	13446.5	16628.8	12600.8	8550.8
Repayments (US$m)	11610.4	12289.4	12720.9	11742.9	0.0	0.0	0.0
Interest (US$m)	8249.8	8612.6	8747.3	7305.0	0.0	0.0	0.0

a. Ranges that reflect the base-case (i.e., most likely) scenario. For IDA countries, planned commitments are not presented by FY but as a three-year-total range; the figures are shown in brackets. A footnote indicates if the pattern of IDA lending has unusual characteristics (e.g., a high degree of frontloading, backloading, or lumpiness). For blend countries, planned IBRD and IDA commitments are presented for each year as a combined total.

b. For future lending, rounded to nearest 0 or 5%. To convey the country strategy more clearly, staff may aggregate sectors.

c. Structural adjustment loans, sector adjustment loans, and debt service reduction loans.

Note: Disbursement data is updated at the end of the first week of the month.

Table E.2 Status of Bank Group Operations in HNP: IBRD Loans and IDA Credits in the Operations Portfolio

Project ID	Fiscal Year	Country	Project Name	Total Project Cost	Original Amount in US$ millions: IBRD	IDA	Cancellations	Undisbursed	Difference between Expected and Actual Disbursements[a]	Environment Category[b]	Development Objectives	Implementation Progress	Elapsed Time between Approval and Effectiveness	Elapsed Time between Initial EPS and Board Approval
Number of closed projects: 94														
Active Projects														
AL-PE-8253	1995	Albania	Health Service Rehabilitation	14.50		12.40		8.76	2.15	C	S	S	3	32
AO-PE-48	1993	Angola	Health	22.20		19.90		14.74	12.70	T	U	S	7	38
AR-PE-43418	1997	Argentina	AIDS Prevention & STD Control	30.00	15.00			15.00		C			..	15
AR-PE-6059	1997	Argentina	Maternal Child Health II	171.00	100.00			100.00		B			..	8
AR-PE-45687	1996	Argentina	Health Insurance Task	29.80	25.00			16.97	-0.33	C	HS	S	3	12
AR-PE-40909	1996	Argentina	Health Insurance Reform	1500.00	350.00			200.00	13.62	C	HS	S	..	12
AR-PE-6030	1996	Argentina	Health Sector Development	144.00	101.40			96.43	17.63	B	HS	S	7	24
AR-PE-6025	1994	Argentina	Maternal Child Health & Nutrition	160.00	100.00			48.22	22.78	C	S	S	2	19
BA-PE-44522	1997	Bosnia-Herzegovina	Essential Hospital Service	33.50		15.00		14.47	2.76	C	S	S	3	9
BA-PE-44424	1996	Bosnia-Herzegovina	War Victims	30.00		5.00		4.87	3.07	C	S	S	2	6
BD-PE-9496	1995	Bangladesh	Nutrition	67.30		59.80		54.21	4.96	C	S	S	2	61
BD-PE-9529	1991	Bangladesh	Population & Health	600.00		180.00		47.63	37.74	C	S	S	9	32
BF-PE-308	1994	Burkina Faso	Population/AIDS Control	23.40		26.30		21.60	3.92	T	S	S	12	17
BF-PE-287	1994	Burkina Faso	Health/Nutrition	40.50		29.20		22.44	3.09	C	S	S	14	84
BG-PE-8318	1996	Bulgaria	Health Sector Restructure	47.10	26.00			25.96	6.03	C	S	S	7	37
BI-PE-216	1995	Burundi	Health/Population II	36.70		21.30		18.95	4.35	C	S	S	9	85
BJ-PE-118	1995	Benin	Population & Health	34.10		27.80		24.12	7.95	C	S	S	14	35
BJ-PE-98	1989	Benin	Health Services Development	32.00		18.60		4.76	3.27	C	S	U	7	31
BO-PE-6166	1990	Bolivia	Integrated Health Development	40.00		20.00		5.23	2.94	C	S	S	7	27
BR-PE-6554	1996	Brazil	Health Sector Reform	750.00	300.00			272.75	16.09	B	S	S	6	12
BR-PE-6546	1994	Brazil	AIDS Control	250.00	160.00			38.92	0.27	C	S	HS	7	17
BR-PE-6403	1990	Brazil	NE Basic Health Service II	610.60	267.00		50.00	27.95	77.95	T	S	S	13	33
CI-PE-1214	1996	Cote d'Ivoire	Population, Health and Nutrition	51.00		40.00		37.08	1.29	C	U	U	6	20
CL-PE-6639	1993	Chile	Health Sector	298.80	90.00			43.29	35.83	B	S	S	3	28
CL-PE-6672	1992	Chile	Technical Assistant & Rehabilitation	45.30	27.00			3.25	3.25	C	S	S	4	9
CM-PE-411	1995	Cameroon	Health/Fertilization/Nutrition	48.08		43.00		38.58	12.45	C	S	U	10	57
CN-PE-3589	1996	China	Disease Prevention	200.00		100.00		87.76	22.40	C	S	S	6	13
CN-PE-37156	1995	China	Iodine Deficiency Disorder	330.00	7.00	20.00		20.95	16.00	C	S	S	10	30
CN-PE-3634	1995	China	Maternal Child Health	138.70		90.00		43.43	5.13	T	HS	HS	3	22
CN-PE-3502	1994	China	Rural Health Manpower	192.00		110.00		58.02	24.33	C	S	U	3	42
CN-PE-3624	1992	China	Infectious Diseases	271.00		129.60		67.85	48.10	C	S	S	4	16
CN-PE-3483	1989	China	Health Services	113.00		52.00		0.17	-3.53	C	S	S	8	27
CO-PE-6854	1993	Colombia	Municipal; Health Service	100.00	50.00			42.87	23.02	C	S	U	7	72
CR-PE-6954	1994	Costa Rica	Health Sector Reform	50.00	22.00			16.81	11.27	C	S	S	18	21
EC-PE-7087	1993	Ecuador	Social Development II/Health & Nutrition	102.20	70.00			38.04	19.19	C	U	U	10	16
EE-PE-8402	1995	Estonia	Health	34.50	18.00			17.37	7.21	C	S	S	6	15
EG-PE-5163	1996	Egypt	Population	19.35		17.20		16.56	1.54	C	S	U	..	17
EG-PE-5152	1992	Egypt	Schistosomiasis Control	44.70		26.84		22.55	13.69	C	S	S	12	32

ET-PE-711	1988	Ethiopia	Family Health	49.60		33.00		10.85	10.48	.	S	S	9	21
GE-PE-8414	1996	Georgia	Health	19.70		14.00		12.73	0.89	C	S	S	4	15
GH-PE-897	1991	Ghana	Health & Population II	34.40		27.00		2.66	1.49	C	S	S	6	45
GM-PE-822	1990	Gambia, The	Women in Development	15.10		7.00		1.13	0.45	C	S	U	7	31
GN-PE-1070	1994	Guinea	Health/Nutrition Sector	27.30		24.60		18.27	2.24	C	S	U	9	44
GQ-PE-649	1992	Equatorial Guinea	Health Improvement Plan	6.00		5.50		1.99	1.86	C	S	U	6	47
GW-PE-1002	1993	Guinea-Bissau	Social	13.00		8.80		2.93	2.41	C	S	S	5	35
GZ-SF-35996	1995	Occupied Territories	Education & Health Rehabilitation	20.00					10.67	.	S	U	3	7
HN-PE-7392	1993	Honduras	Nutrition/Health	54.20		25.00		3.96	3.03	C	S	S	8	16
HR-PE-39450	1995	Croatia	Health Project	40.00	40.00			13.73	13.73	C	HS	HS	6	5
HT-PE-7311	1990	Haiti	Health & Population	33.70		28.20		22.09	19.07	C	U	S	5	27
HU-PE-8484	1993	Hungary	Health Services	132.60	91.00			69.03	45.33	C	U	U	6	19
ID-PE-42540	1997	Indonesia	Iodine Deficiency Control	45.30	28.50			27.50	-0.50	C	S	S	2	15
ID-PE-41896	1996	Indonesia	Capacity Building	25.00	20.00			19.41	1.26	C	S	U	4	10
ID-PE-39643	1996	Indonesia	Sexually Transmitted Diseases/AIDS	35.20	24.80			24.07	7.02	C	S	S	3	13
ID-PE-3965	1995	Indonesia	Health IV: Improving Health	276.00	88.00			82.41	-5.49	C	S	S	3	35
ID-PE-3914	1993	Indonesia	Health	164.10	93.50			37.37	5.21	C	S	S	7	71
IN-PE-44449	1997	India	Rural Women Development	53.50		19.50		18.79		C			..	13
IN-PE-10531	1997	India	Reproductive Health	309.00		248.30		249.80		T			..	24
IN-PE-10511	1997	India	Malaria Control	170.00		164.80		164.80		B			..	20
IN-PE-10473	1997	India	Tuberculosis Control	142.40		142.40		136.94	2.32	T	S	S	4	41
IN-PE-35825	1996	India	State Health System II	425.00		350.00		315.56	12.01	C	S	S	3	14
IN-PE-10489	1995	India	Health	158.90		133.00		117.23	18.24	T	S	S	3	18
IN-PE-10457	1994	India	Population IX	130.00		88.60		75.72	11.99	T	S	S	3	22
IN-PE-10455	1994	India	Blindness Control	137.80		117.80		101.17	19.43	C	S	S	8	22
IN-PE-10424	1993	India	National Leprosy Elimination	135.50		85.00		59.20	35.46	C	S	S	9	17
IN-PE-9977	1993	India	ICDS II	248.80		194.00		171.67	72.26	C	S	S	6	51
IN-PE-10393	1992	India	AIDS Prevention	99.60		84.00		32.07	29.76	C	S	S	6	7
IN-PE-9963	1992	India	Population VIII	88.00		79.00		71.38	44.97	C	S	S	23	30
IN-PE-10361	1991	India	ICDS I	315.00	10.00	96.00	31.65	22.42	44.18	T	S	S	4	29
IN-PE-9940	1990	India	Population Training	313.40	10.00	86.70	32.74	8.69	37.34	C	S	S	10	17
IN-PE-9932	1990	India	Nutrition	139.10		95.80	29.81	3.49	22.87	C	S	S	6	26
IR-PE-5222	1993	Iran, Islamic Rep. of	Health & Family Planning	294.00	141.40			105.03	80.27	T	S	S	1	9
JO-PE-5319	1993	Jordan	Health II	30.00	20.00			18.48	6.18	C	S	U	12	44
KE-PE-1333	1995	Kenya	Sexually Transmitted Diseases	95.00		40.00		33.75	7.45	C	S	S	5	15
KE-PE-1339	1992	Kenya	Health Rehabilitation	34.00		31.00		18.91	18.94	C	S	U	8	47
KE-PE-1312	1990	Kenya	Population IV	37.00		35.00		26.80	24.63	C	S	U	6	10
KG-PE-8523	1996	Kyrgyz Republic	Health	20.10		18.50		16.52	-0.11	C	S	S	5	25
KH-PE-4034	1997	Cambodia	Disease Control & Health	35.60		30.40		28.67	2.80	T	S	S	..	13
KM-PE-596	1994	Comoros	Population & Human Resources	16.00		13.00		4.48	0.97	B	HS	HS	6	38
LA-PE-4200	1995	Lao Peoples Dem. Rep.	Health System Reform	24.00		19.20		15.90	2.43	C	S	S	5	71
LB-PE-34004	1995	Lebanon	Health Project	35.70	35.70			34.75	13.34	T	S	U	10	13
LK-PE-10526	1997	Sri Lanka	Health Services Development	22.60		18.80		18.09	1.25	C	S	S	3	28
LS-PE-1395	1990	Lesotho	Health/Population II	21.50		12.10		3.83	2.81	T	S	S	4	32
MA-PE-42415	1996	Morocco	Health	6865.00	68.00			68.00	1.50	C	S	S	7	39
MA-PE-5440	1990	Morocco	Health Sector Investment	171.30	104.00			16.75	16.75	C	S	S	7	18
MG-PE-1520	1991	Madagascar	National Health Sector	42.50		31.00		9.65	7.69	C	S	S	11	49
MK-PE-36089	1996	FYR Macedonia	Health Sector Transition	19.40		16.90		16.18	5.06	C	S	S	6	21
ML-PE-1727	1991	Mali	Health/Population	61.40		26.60		6.07	3.89	B	HS	S	12	54
MR-PE-1855	1992	Mauritania	Health/Population	24.40		15.70		3.51	1.45	C	S	S	7	56

(Table continues on the following page.)

Table E.2 (*continued*)

Project ID	Fiscal Year	Country	Project Name	Total Project Cost	Original Amount in US$ millions: IBRD	IDA	Cancel-lations	Undis-bursed	Difference between Expected and Actual Disburse-ments[a]	Environ-ment Category[b]	Develop-ment Objectives	Imple-mentation Progress	Elapsed Time between Approval and Effective-ness	Elapsed Time between Initial EPS and Board Approval
MW-PE-1646	1991	Malawi	Health, Nutrition & Population Sector Credit	73.60		55.50		33.05	34.42	C	S	S	3	37
MX-PE-7689	1996	Mexico	Basic Health II	443.40	310.00			287.81	15.65	C	S	S	6	18
MY-PE-4312	1994	Malaysia	Health	101.30	50.00			38.94	10.28	C	S	S	2	44
MZ-PE-1792	1996	Mozambique	Health Sector Recovery	355.70		98.70		87.63	17.94	C	S	S	5	74
MZ-PE-1801	1993	Mozambique	Food Security	8.10		6.30		4.08	2.96	T	S	S	10	18
MZ-PE-1787	1989	Mozambique	Health & Nutrition	42.50		27.00		1.35	-28.89	C	S	S	7	14
NE-PE-1999	1997	Niger	Health II	50.00		40.00		38.83	0.57	C			..	29
NE-PE-1976	1992	Niger	Population	24.10		17.60		7.91	5.99	C	S	S	8	60
NG-PE-2106	1991	Nigeria	Health Fund	94.50	70.00		16.00	38.66	49.06	C	S	S	10	40
NG-PE-2094	1991	Nigeria	Population	93.50		78.50		66.41	50.69	C	S	U	9	49
NG-PE-2125	1990	Nigeria	National Drugs	85.10	68.10		16.20	22.31	35.36	C	S	U	11	33
NG-PE-2091	1989	Nigeria	Health & Population	36.80	27.60		11.74	4.98	16.72	C	S	U	9	28
NI-PE-7778	1994	Nicaragua	Health Sector Project	20.00		15.00		5.40	2.09	B	HS	S	3	20
NP-PE-10460	1994	Nepal	Population & Health	39.00		26.70		24.66	11.53	C	S	S	3	59
PA-PE-7846	1995	Panama	Rural Health	50.00	25.00			22.96	12.96	C	S	S	8	25
PE-PE-8048	1994	Peru	Basic Health/Nutrition	42.00	34.00			24.11	11.55	C	S	S	4	24
PG-PE-4399	1993	Papua New Guinea	Population Project	32.70	6.90			5.84	3.88	C	S	U	8	19
PH-PE-4567	1995	Philippines	Women's Health & Safe Motherhood	136.40	18.00			17.62	1.66	C	S	S	4	36
PH-PE-4568	1993	Philippines	Urban Health & Nutrition	82.20		70.00		59.67	17.94	C	S	S	10	36
PH-PE-4518	1989	Philippines	Health Development	108.40	70.10			2.50	2.50	C	S	S	7	30
PK-PE-37827	1996	Pakistan	Northern Health	57.70		26.70		25.61	2.66	C	S	S	..	20
PK-PE-10492	1995	Pakistan	Population Welfare	65.10		65.10		56.04	9.47	C	S	S	4	23
PK-PE-10414	1993	Pakistan	Family Health II	114.00		48.00		37.73	15.93	C	S	S	5	26
PK-PE-10371	1991	Pakistan	Family Health	62.90		45.00		31.15	20.78	C	U	U	10	51
PL-PE-8587	1992	Poland	Health	205.00	130.00		30.00	53.72	61.86	C	S	S	8	20
PY-PE-7927	1997	Paraguay	Mental Health/Child Development	62.40	21.80			21.22	0.17	C	S	S	5	23
RO-PE-8759	1992	Romania	Health Service Rehabilitation	210.40	150.00			55.70	55.70	C	S	U	3	10
RU-PE-8814	1997	Russia	Health Reform Pilot	98.40	66.00			66.00		C			..	51
RU-PE-38571	1996	Russia	Medical Equipment	305.00	270.00			252.18	-9.48	C	S	S	7	18
RW-PE-2237	1991	Rwanda	Health & Population	26.00		19.60		16.88	15.76	C	S	S	12	53
RY-PE-5910	1993	Yemen, Republic of	Family Health	30.20		26.60		23.74	14.69	C	S	U	15	12
RY-PE-5822	1990	Yemen, Republic of	Health Sector Development	19.10		15.00		10.49	9.08	C	S	S	14	8
SL-PE-2422	1996	Sierra Leone	Health Sector	20.00		20.00		17.69	0.73	C	U	U	6	31
SN-PE-41567	1997	Senegal	Endemic Diseases	19.00		14.90		15.03		C			..	16
SN-PE-35615	1995	Senegal	Community Nutrition	18.20		18.20		14.05	6.45	C	HS	S	7	14
ST-PE-2542	1992	Sao Tome and Principe	Health & Nutrition	12.00		11.40		5.89	4.94	C	S	S	10	21
TD-PE-35601	1995	Chad	Population & AIDS Control	26.10		20.40		15.87	-1.05	C	S	S	6	13
TD-PE-509	1994	Chad	Health & Safe Motherhood	30.00		18.50		8.08	-2.45	C	S	S	8	33
TD-PE-520	1990	Chad	Social Development Program	53.80		23.20		1.89	-15.05	B	S	S	10	23
TN-PE-5738	1991	Tunisia	Hospital Management	49.50	30.00			16.34	16.21	T	S	S	10	9
TN-PE-5717	1991	Tunisia	Population & Family	63.20	26.00			3.95	3.95	C	HS	S	7	14

TR-PE-9076	1995	Turkey	Health II	200.00	150.00			136.17	49.82	C	S	S	4	70
TR-PE-9030	1989	Turkey	Health I	146.30	75.00			27.16	26.01	C	HS	HS	17	35
TZ-PE-2774	1990	Tanzania	Health & Nutrition	70.00		47.60		24.00	20.47	C	S	U	1	26
UG-PE-2971	1995	Uganda	District Health	63.00		45.00		37.30	1.70	C	U	U	5	19
UG-PE-2963	1994	Uganda	Sexual Transmission Intervention	70.00		50.00		40.41	9.76	C	U	U	3	58
UY-PE-8161	1995	Uruguay	Health Sector Development	28.00	15.60			13.55	4.97	C	U	U	4	27
VE-PE-8215	1995	Venezuela	Health Service Reform	108.00	54.00			51.72	15.89	B	S	S	14	32
VE-PE-8227	1993	Venezuela	Endemic Disease Control	188.00	94.00		20.00	47.17	51.84	B	S	S	15	17
VE-PE-8204	1991	Venezuela	Social Development	320.90	100.00		15.00	52.44	67.44	C	S	U	10	16
VN-PE-4841	1996	Viet Nam	Population & Family	133.00		50.00		45.83	3.13	C	S	U	4	24
VN-PE-4838	1996	Viet Nam	National Health Support	127.20		101.20		93.19	3.03	C	S	S	4	51
ZM-PE-3239	1995	Zambia	Health Sector	557.00		56.00		46.78	10.53	C	S	S	3	18
ZW-PE-3333	1993	Zimbabwe	Sexual Transmission Intervention	87.30		64.50		34.34	9.40	T	S	S	3	8
ZW-PE-3302	1991	Zimbabwe	Family Health II	117.00	25.00			6.27	6.27	C	S	S	8	42
TOTAL				24,095.03	4,390.40	4,752.34	253.14	6,183.29	1,916.86					

	Active Projects	*Closed Projects*	*Total*
Total disbursed (IBRD and IDA)	2,691.89	2,683.21	5,375.10
Of which repaid	121.77	577.87	699.64
Total now held by IBRD and IDA	8,787.80	1,982.71	10,770.51
Amount sold	0.00	7.95	7.95
Of which repaid	0.00	7.95	7.95
Total undisbursed	6,183.27	20.53	6,203.80

a. Intended disbursements to date minus actual disbursements to date as projected at appraisal.
b. The environment assessement category list is as follows:
A: Full environmental assessment required
B: Partial environmental assessment required
C: None required
D: Free-standing environmental project
T: To be decided
c. Following the FY94 Annual Review of Portfolio Performance (ARPP), a letter-based system was introduced (HS=highly satisfactory, S=satisfactory, U=unstatisfactory, HU=highly unsatisfactory); see Proposed Improvements in Project and Portfolio Performance Rating Methodology(SecM94-901), August 23, 1994.

Note: Disbursement data is updated at the end of the first week of the month.
.. indicates data not available.

Status of Bank Group Operations in HNP, 1997: IBRD Loans and IDA Credits in the Operations Portfolio

Project ID	*Fiscal Year*	*Country*	*Project Name*	*Project Cost US$m*	*Amount US$M*
1999	1997	Niger	Health II	50.0	40.0
4034	1997	Cambodia	Disease Control & Health	35.6	30.4
6059	1997	Argentina	Mental Child Health 2	171.0	100.0
7927	1997	Paraguay	Mental Health/Child Develoment	31.2	21.8
8814	1997	Russia	Health	100.1	70.0
9095	1997	Turkey	Primary Health Care Services	200.0	15.0
10473	1997	India	Tuberculosis Control	142.4	142.4
10511	1997	India	Malaria Control	203.9	164.8
10526	1997	Sri Lanka	Health Services Development	22.6	18.8
10531	1997	India	Reproductive Health 1	309.0	248.3
36956	1997	Indonesia	Safe Motherhood	40.0	40.0
41567	1997	Senegal	Endemic Diseases	19.0	14.9
42540	1997	Indonesia	Iodine Deficiency Control	45.3	28.5
43418	1997	Argentina	AIDS Prevention & STD Control	30.0	15.0
44449	1997	India	Rural Women's Development	53.5	19.5
44522	1997	Bosnia-Herzegovina	Essential Hospital Services	33.5	15.0
TOTAL	1997			1487.1	984.4

FY98 to FY2000 Pipeline	*Number of Projects*	*Amount US$m*	*Discounted by 35% Amount US$m*
Estimated FY98 Pipeline	27	1,260.1	819.1
Estimated FY99 Pipeline	42	2,955.2	1,920.9
Estimated FY00 Pipeline	40	3,033.6	1,971.8

Table E.3 IFC and MIGA HNP Program, FY 1994–1996

	Past		
Category	*FY94*	*FY95*	*FY96*
IFC approvals (US$m)	61	30	1
Sector (%)			
Financial Services	100	100	100
TOTAL	100	100	100
Investment instrument (%)			
Loans	0	0	0
Equity	100	67	100
Quasi-equity[a]	0	33	0
Other	0	0	0
TOTAL	100	100	100
MIGA guarantees (US$m)	..	..	..
MIGA commitments (US$m)	..	..	..

a. Includes quasi-equity types of both loan and equity instruments.

Note: .. indicates data not available.

Table E.4 Summary of Economic and Sector Work
(US$ thousands)

Category	*Last Fiscal Year Annual*	*FY97*	*FY98*	*FY99*
Agriculture	6,445	6,179	5,332	171
Education	3,279	2,347	2,075	144
Electric Power & Energy	957	1,139	935	120
Environment	4,060	4,143	1,324	30
Finance	4,119	3,233	2,359	0
Human Resources	5	5	8	0
Industry	904	486	461	0
Mining	0	31	71	0
Multisector	17,453	14,535	16,496	658
Oil & Gas	2,011	1,752	699	386
Population, Health, Nutrition	3,867	3,239	1,821	252
Public Sector Management	7,762	4,862	4,107	275
Social Sector	5,338	3,964	3,078	410
Telecommunications	394	262	79	19
Transportation	3,208	1,486	672	98
Unidentified	14,213	13,472	8,223	1,363
Urban Development	1,204	1,228	1,056	79
Water Supply & Sanitation	1,321	821	682	0
TOTAL	76,537	63,183	49,476	4,004

Ongoing and Planned HNP Economic and Sector Work, FY 1997–1999

Project ID	*Fiscal Year*	*Country*	*Project Name*	*Final Cover*	*$ Amount (thousands)*
12930	1997	Mauritius	Health Sector Review	White	
15026	1997	Africa Region	Gender Action Plan	Green	
15837	1997	Bangladesh	Population & Health Sector Strategy.		
16219	1997	India	State Health Reform		
19389	1997	Azerbaijan	Poverty Assessment	Gray	
19390	1997	Azerbaijan	Azerbaijan Health Note	White	
36239	1997	Djibouti	Poverty Assessment	Green	
36484	1997	Kazakstan	Health Sector Note	White	
36485	1997	Tajikistan	Health Sector Note	White	
36610	1997	Costa Rica	Poverty Assessment	Gray	
37171	1997	Asia Region	Health Reform in Asia	Yellow	
38950	1997	Argentina	Health Financing	Gray	
42453	1997	Russia	Health Sector Note	White	
43186	1997	Ghana	Gender Strategy	White	
44882	1997	Pakistan	Health Strategy		
45042	1997	Philippines	Environmental Health Assessment		
49394	1997	Russia	Social Challenges	White	
49444	1997	Indonesia	Pharmaceuticals		
49445	1997	Indonesia	Health Patterns		
49446	1997	Indonesia	Health Financing		
49519	1997	El Salvador	Rural Health Care	Green	
Estimated Number of Reports:	1996				3,867
Estimated Number of Reports:	1997	21			3,239
Estimated Number of Reports:	1998	15			1,821
Estimated Number of Reports:	1999	23			252

Table E.5 HNP Sector: Selected Indicators of Bank Portfolio Performance and Management

Indicator	*FY94*	*FY95*	*FY96*	*FY97*
Portfolio Performance				
Number of projects under implementation	122	139	154	151
Average implementation period (years)[a]	4	4	4	4
Percent of problem projects rated U or HU[b] (for past years, rated 3 or 4)				
Development objectives[c]	12	7	8	7
Implementation progress (or overall status for past years)[d]	20	15	15	21
Canceled during FY in US$m	80	129	52	75
Disbursement ratio (%)[e]	13	16	16	14
Disbursement lag (%)[f]	41	37	34	33
Portfolio Management				
Supervision resources (total US$ thousands)	7,377	6,617	7,467	11,100
Average supervision (US$ thousands/project)	60	48	48	74
Supervision resources by location (in %)				
Percent headquarters	0	0	56	51
Percent resident mission	0	0	44	49
Supervision resources by rating category (US$ thousands/project)				
Projects rated HS or S	62	47	48	74
Projects rated U or HU	57	50	53	80

a. Average age of projects in the Bank's country portfolio.

b. Rating scale: "HS" denotes highly satisfactory, "S" denotes satisfactory, "U" denotes unsatisfactory, and "HU" denotes highly unsatisfactory.

c. Extent to which the project will meet its development objectives (see OD 13.05, Annex D2, Preparation of Implementation Summary [Form 590]).

d. Assessment of overall performance of the project based on the ratings given to individual aspects of project implementation (e.g., management, availability of funds, compliance with legal covenants) and to development objectives (see OD 13.05, Annex D2, Preparation of Implementation Summary [Form 590]). The overall status is not given a better rating than that given to project development objectives.

e. Ratio of disbursements during the year to the undisbursed balance of the Bank's portfolio at the beginning of the year: investment projects only.

f. For all projects comprising the Bank's country portfolio, the percentage difference between actual cumulative disbursements and the cumulative disbursement estimates as given in the "Original SAR/PR Forecast" or, if the loan amounts have been modified, in the "Revised Forecast." The country portfolio disbursement lag is effectively the weighted average of disbursement lags for projects comprising the Bank's country portfolio, where the weights used are the respective project shares in the total cumulative disbursement estimates.

Note: Disbursement data is updated at the end of the first week of the month. Supervision resources include Salaries, Benefits, and Travel for all sources of funds but excludes FAO staff and PCR task costs.

ANNEX F

HNP Sector Strategy Matrix (FY 1998–2000)

HNP Sector Strategy Matrix (FY 1998–2000)

Underlying HNP Issues	*Development Objectives*	*Bank's HNP Sector Strategy*	*Progress Indicators (See Annexes B to E)*	***Bank Instruments*** *Lending/ Credits*	*Non-Lending*	*Other Partners*
A. SHARPENING STRATEGIC POLICY DIRECTIONS						
900 million of 1.3 billion poor without access to basic health care 2 million deaths annually due to vaccine-preventable diseases 200 million children under 5 who suffer from malnutrition and anemia 120 million couples without family planning and 8.1 million maternal and perinatal deaths annually 30 percent of world without access to safe water and sanitation systems	*Improve the health, nutrition and population outcomes of the world's poor, and protect other segments of the population from the impoverishing effects of illness* by: • targeting of low income groups, geographic locations, and poverty-related diseases, and services used by the poor • expanding equitable access to basic health services • maintaining policy oversight in intersectoral areas such as rural and urban development, social policy, education, agriculture, and environment	Work closely with governments to encourage them to provide, or mandate, affordable & cost-effective services for the poor: • basic immunization • management of sick child • maternal & perinatal care • family planning • targeted nutrition • school health • communicable disease control Work with other sectors to ensure healthy intersectoral policies such as tobacco & alcohol control and taxation, appropriate food subsidies, road safety, & environmental issues	*Health Indicators* • life expectancy • infant and under-5 mortality • adult mortality • tobacco attributable illness *Nutrition Indicators* • low birth weight • child malnutrition • anemia • obesity *Maternal and Reproductive Health* • fertility • maternal mortality *Health Services* • access to basic care • immunization coverage	FY98-00 Increase IDA and IBRD loans for targeted programs for the poor Increase use of fiscal instruments (tobacco, alcohol tax, etc.)	FY98-00 CAS & partner dialogue Annual status rep FY98 Regional strategies FY99 Country strategies	WHO, UNICEF, UNFPA, UNDP, UNAIDS, FAO, ILO, regional banks, bilaterals, NGOs, & private sector
Inadequate action by governments in providing public health services (underfinanced, low quality, poorly managed, badly staffed, ill equipped government run services). Poorly regulated private sector leading to excess profit taking, problems with quality control, ineffective care, low coverage, and inadequate risk pooling Pervasive patient dissatisfaction	*Enhance the performance of health care systems* by: • improving public services (ensuring equitable access to preventive and curative health services that are affordable, cost-effective, efficient, of good quality, responsive to consumer choice); • harnessing non-governmental resources more effectively (regulations, increased quality monitoring, licensing)	Work closely with governments, NGOs, and civil society to: • strengthen policy making, governance, accountability, management, and monitoring and evaluation • provide incentives for public and private sectors to improve efficiency, effectiveness, and quality through competition • foster partnerships with non-governmental providers • conduct consumer surveys	New indicators are needed in the following areas: • policymaking, governance, and management capacity • access to health care • utilization and demand • efficiency and effectiveness • quality control • public and private providers • consumer satisfaction • regulatory systems	FY98-00 Use of micro and mini loans to pilot new lending Increase in sector-wide projects Use SECALs	FY98-00 CAS and partner dialogue FY98-99 OED and other studies Develop indicators	WHO, national agencies, academic institutes, and private sector OED, DEC, IFC, PSD, and others
Low- and middle-income countries consume US$250 billion in health care (4 % of their GDP) 44 low-income countries do not have adequate financial resources to pay the needed US$10–US$20 per capita for essential services Some middle-income countries have uncontrolled cost escalation	*Secure sustainable health care financing* by • mobilizing adequate levels of health financing through broad-based risk pooling • maintaining effective public and private expenditure control • developing improved budget allocation processes at the national and local levels	Work closely with governments to: • strengthen their policymaking role and direct involvement in health care financing, especially in countries where health care expenditure is less than 3 % or greater than 7 % of GDP • use national health accounts and other relevant data in policymaking processes	*Coverage Through Risk-Pooling* • percentage of total population *Source of Financing* • general revenues • social & private insurance • user charges • foreign aid *Expenditure categories* • by expenditure and service • by public and private provider • by recurrent expenditure	Use of micro and mini loans to pilot new lending Increase health financing projects Use SECALs	FY98-00 CAS and partner dialogue *Annually* Country and global exp. reviews	WHO, national agencies, academic institutes, country debts, IMF

B. ACHIEVING GREATER DEVELOPMENT IMPACT					
Human development (HNP, education, and social protection strategies) often poorly reflected in CASs, CEM, and other documents, and discussed only at low levels	*Maximize policy impact*	Focus attention on HNP priority areas in ESW, CAS, and lending Elevate discussion on key HNP issues to macro-level	Incr. inclusion of HNP priorities in CASs, ESW, and lending operations Incr. inclusion of HNP priorities in high-level country discussions	FY98-00 Annual status reports	Country units, IMF, DEC
Drop in admin. budget for ESW and unfocused research Inadequate supervision of operational research components of projects	*Underpin lending with better analysis and research*	Reverse recent cutbacks for sectoral analyses and link research agenda more closely with operational priority areas in HNP sector Improve quality in design and supervision of operational research	Incr. allocation of administrative budget for ESW, research, and learning about HNP priority areas Incr. consultation with technically competent staff during design and supervision of operational research	FY98-00 Annual status reports	Country units, DEC
Unfocused portfolio (questionable development impact in some cases) Disproportionate Bank resources spent on non-poor populations Lack of clear commitment to reform by some clients	*Increase selectivity*	Apply selectivity according to: • the degree of consistency with HNP policy objectives and potential development impact • impact on HNP outcomes for large populations of the poor • commitment by clients to significant reform	Incr. ESW and lending focused on HNP priorities Incr. ESW and lending in countries with large poor population groups Decr. lending in countries with lack of commitment to reform	FY98-00 Annual status reports	Country units
Rapidly expanding underlying knowledge base, but which is often paper-based, disorganized, and inaccessible Findings by OED, QAG, and other groups often not implemented Narrow range of instruments used Rigid application of business processes Insensitivity and unresponsiveness to client needs often leads to lack of client satisfaction	*Improve quality of client services*	Develop and maintain user-friendly knowledge base in priority areas Improve performance by applying lessons learned, strengthening quality at entry, and improving supervision of existing projects Use broader range of instruments (see attachment on sector wide approaches and new instruments) Streamline business processes and procurement procedures to HNP Conduct client satisfaction surveys	Availability of help desks, on-line database of reference and statistical material, and knowledge base of various aspects of HNP systems Improvements in QAG, OED, and other quality ratings Objective assessment of wider application of lending instruments Objective assessment of increased flexibility in business processes and procurement practices Results of client satisfaction survey	FY98-00 Annual status reports External audit	QAG, OED, CODE, EDI
Frequent lack of evidence-based monitoring and evaluation (M&E) criteria	*Strengthen monitoring and evaluation (M&E) of impact*	Develop better M&E indicators Strengthen borrower and Bank capacity and commitment to monitoring and evaluation	Tracking of development indicators Objective assessment of closer links between HNP priority areas, project design, and M&E	FY98-00 Annual status reports	OED, CODE

(Matrix continues on the following page.)

HNP Sector Strategy Matrix (*continued*)

Underlying HNP Issues	*Development Objectives*	*Bank's HNP Sector Strategy*	*Progress Indicators (See Annexes B to E)*	***Bank Instruments*** *Lending/ Credits*	*Non-Lending*	*Other Partners*
C. EMPOWERING STAFF						
Many staff whose skills do not match the HNP sector priorities Low staff-lending ratios in HNP sector compared with Bank-wide norms and skewed distribution across the regions HQ staff are often insensitive to client needs and satisfaction	*Empower staff*	Focus skill-mix, staff policies, and training on priority areas Ensure that staffing ratios in the HNP sector are consistent with Bank-wide norms and that staffing ratios within the HNP sector are realigned according to staff involvement in addressing the three priority areas and relative responsibility for the lending portfolio. Be more responsive to client needs by listening more and getting closer to the client in the field	Objective assessment of skills-mix staff policies and training programs Adjustment in HNP staff according to Bank-wide norms and relative share of lending portfolio. Incr. in number of skilled local resident staff and surveys on client satisfaction		FY98-00 Annual status reports	LLC, EDI
D. STRENGTHENING PARTNERSHIPS						
Limited partnerships with other agencies despite clear increase in international leadership Often clients are left out of the limited collaborative efforts that do exist Limited participation in major international collective initiatives that have a potential dramatic impact on global health	*Enhance partnerships*	Join forces with other agencies through country-level collaboration and in addressing major issues such as vaccination, the HIV/AIDS crisis, emerging drug resistance, and child mortality. Involve clients more substantially in collaborative work Participate in major collective initiatives proposed by the Global Forum on Health Research	Objective assessment of increased partnerships with clients, civil society, stakeholders, and other agencies Objective assessment of client participation in HNP initiatives Participation in one or more major international initiatives	FY98-00 Support through project components	FY98-00 Use of SGP Annual reports	WHO, UNICEF, UNFPA, UNDP, UNAIDS, FAO, ILO, regional banks, bilaterals, NGOs, & private sector

Application of Lending Instruments to HNP Sector

In low-income countries that use IDA credits—when the proposed health, nutrition, and population interventions would contribute significantly to achieving poverty alleviation objectives— the Bank will:[1]

- increase the IDA financing, where necessary, in an effort to ensure that the development objective of the operation is not compromised by lack of counterpart funding;
- mainstream comprehensive financing (recurrent and capital expenditures) for activities supported by the project (i.e., targeted disease control, nutrition, and population programs that specifically benefit the poor);
- avoid a substitution effect by ensuring that Bank resources contribute to a net increase in the resources available to the HNP sector rather than allowing governments to shift their own resources to other areas.

In the case of both IDA credits and IBRD loans—when the main objective of the proposed operation is to improve the performance of health care delivery systems rather than poverty relief—the Bank will:

- use smaller TA loans or *pilot project facilities* (currently being developed by the New Products Committee) to deal specifically with issues relating to enhancing the institutional capacity of governments in meeting their policy making, management, evaluation, regulatory, and financing responsibilities in the HNP sector;
- use a coordinated pipeline of specific investment loans or time-slice sector investment loans to implement programs that have a medium-term time frame for achieving development objectives;
- increase product selectivity through: (i) more emphasis on a few critical activities in the public sector that will facilitate a re-balancing in the role of the state and non-governmental activities in service delivery systems; (ii) on-lending arrangements (subsidiary loan agreements) and a closer partnership with the private sector development and infrastructure branches of the Bank, IFC, and MIGA in facilitating the flow of funds to non-governmental health care delivery systems;[2] and (iii) introduction of mechanisms that will allow clients to apply for financial support from the Bank for a select group of "certified" programs that would be fully developed and implemented by other agencies or the private sector; and
- make more effective use of new lending instruments and sector adjustment loans (SECALs) to support broad sector- wide institutional reforms that have significant transition costs (avoid loading traditional investment loans with complicated conditionalities).[3]

When the main objective is to improve financial sustainability of health systems or introduce tighter expenditure controls that have fiscal implications, a more aggressive strategy will be pursued to:

- conduct detailed analysis of the fiscal implications, public/private affordability, institutional capacity, political commitment, and sustainability of various reform options before proceeding with such operations;[4] and
- include health financing contents, whenever possible, as an integral part of new lending instruments and broader public finance SECALs rather than attempt complicated health financing reforms under investment loans.

Such adjustment operations need to be complemented by direct investment loans that address underlying institutional and management issues.

1. The same recommendations would apply in a modified manner to IBRD loans to middle-income countries where the primary objective is poverty alleviation.

2. A careful financial viability and risk analysis should always be undertaken as part of the project justification for this type of operation.

3. Specific targeted interventions often have a greater impact when underpinned by a combination of broad macroeconomic adjustment operations, public sector reform projects, or sector adjustment loans that address resilient underlying sectoral distortions.

4. This should include detailed economic modeling and projections of existing and alternative policy options.

ANNEX G

World Bank Maps

Fertility Decline, 1980–1995

Progress in Achieving Child Survival Goals, 1990–1995

Child Malnutrition, 1985–1995

Malaria Distribution and Reported Drug Resistance

Health Expenditures as Percent of GDP

Active and Future World Bank/IDA Financed HNP Projects

The World by Region

Fertility Decline, 1980 – 1995

Percent change in the total fertility rate:

- TFR already low in 1980 (<2.3)
- TFR decline of 30% or more
- TFR decline between 10% and 30%
- < 10% decline in TFR
- No data

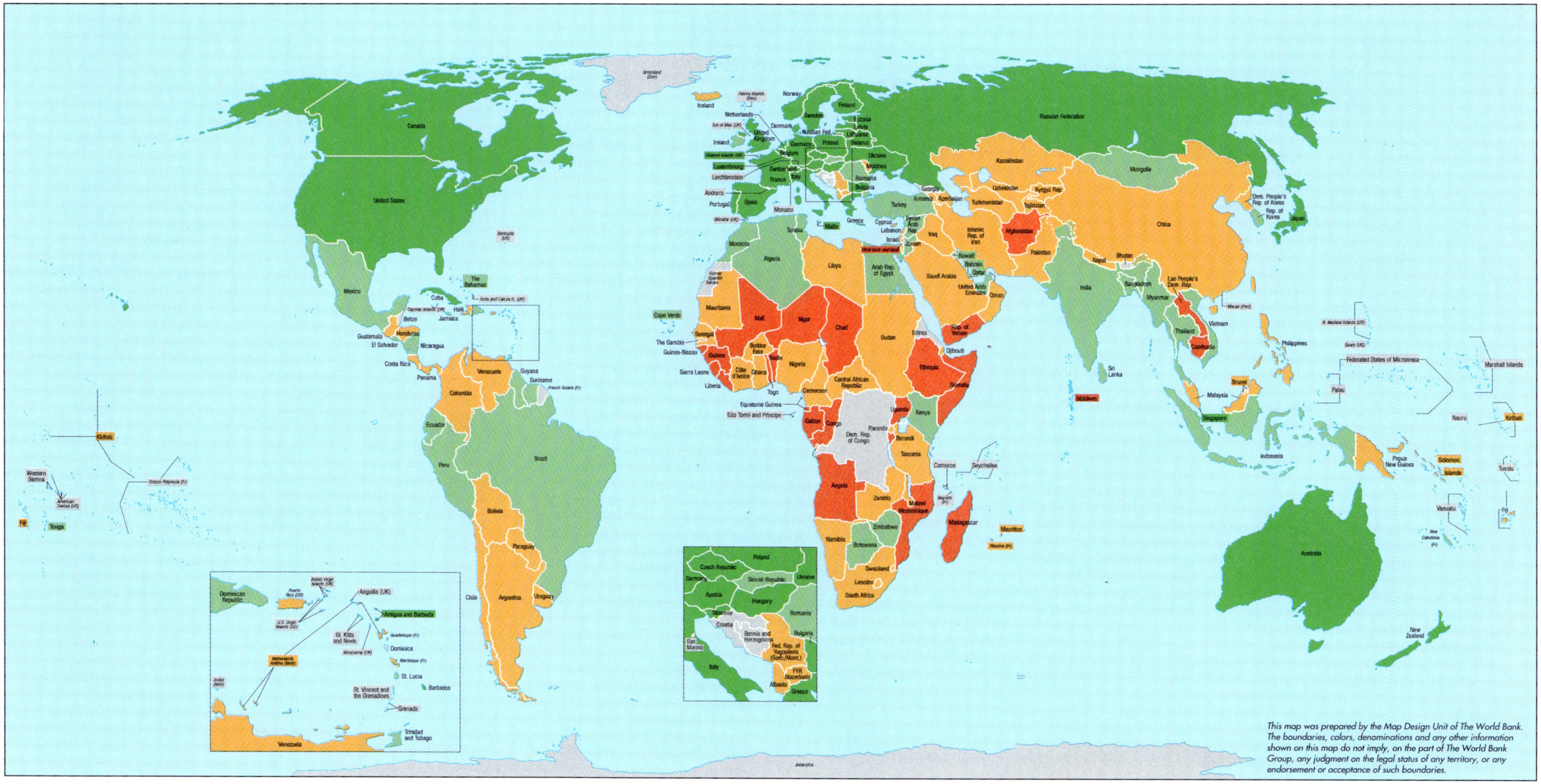

IBRD 28973

AUGUST 1998

Progress in Achieving Child Survival Goals, 1990 – 1995

- Child mortality rate already very low (< 20 per thousand)
- On target to achieve goal of 1/3 reduction in child mortality by the year 2000
- Only slight improvement in child mortality- not on target
- Increased child mortality
- No data

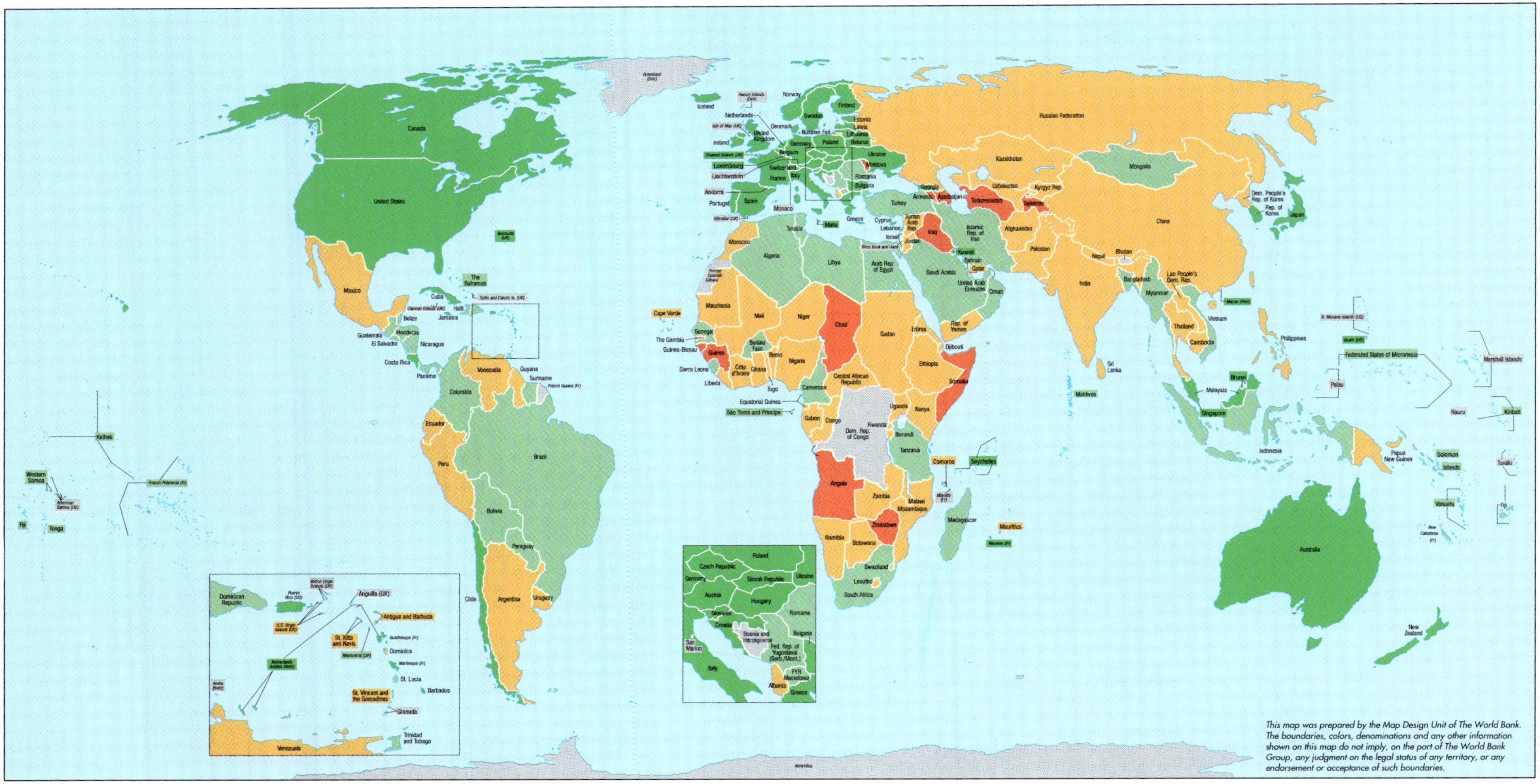

This map was prepared by the Map Design Unit of The World Bank. The boundaries, colors, denominations and any other information shown on this map do not imply, on the part of The World Bank Group, any judgment on the legal status of any territory, or any endorsement or acceptance of such boundaries.

IBRD 28972

AUGUST 1998

Child Malnutrition, 1985 – 1995

Percent of children less than 5 years old who are malnourished:

- Less than 10%
- 10% - 19%
- 20% - 29%
- 30% - 39%
- 40% or more
- No data

IBRD 28974

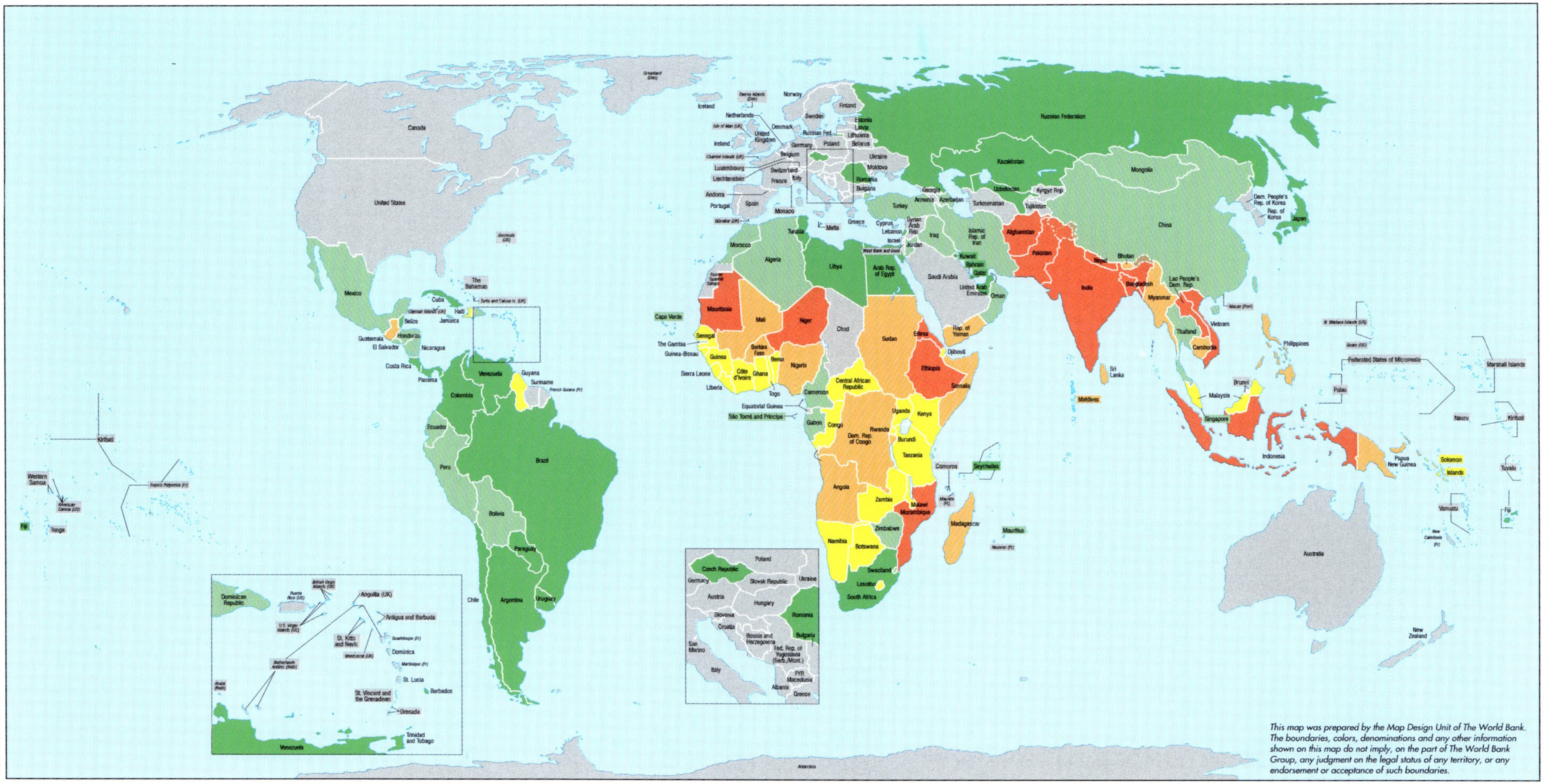

This map was prepared by the Map Design Unit of The World Bank. The boundaries, colors, denominations and any other information shown on this map do not imply, on the part of The World Bank Group, any judgment on the legal status of any territory, or any endorsement or acceptance of such boundaries.

AUGUST 1998

Malaria Distribution and Reported Drug Resistance

- 90% of malaria incidence and death
- Remaining malaria incidence and death
- Chloroquine resistance
- Sulfadoxine-Pyrimethamine (Fansidar) resistance
- Multi-drug resistance

Chloroquine and Fansidar resistance widespread

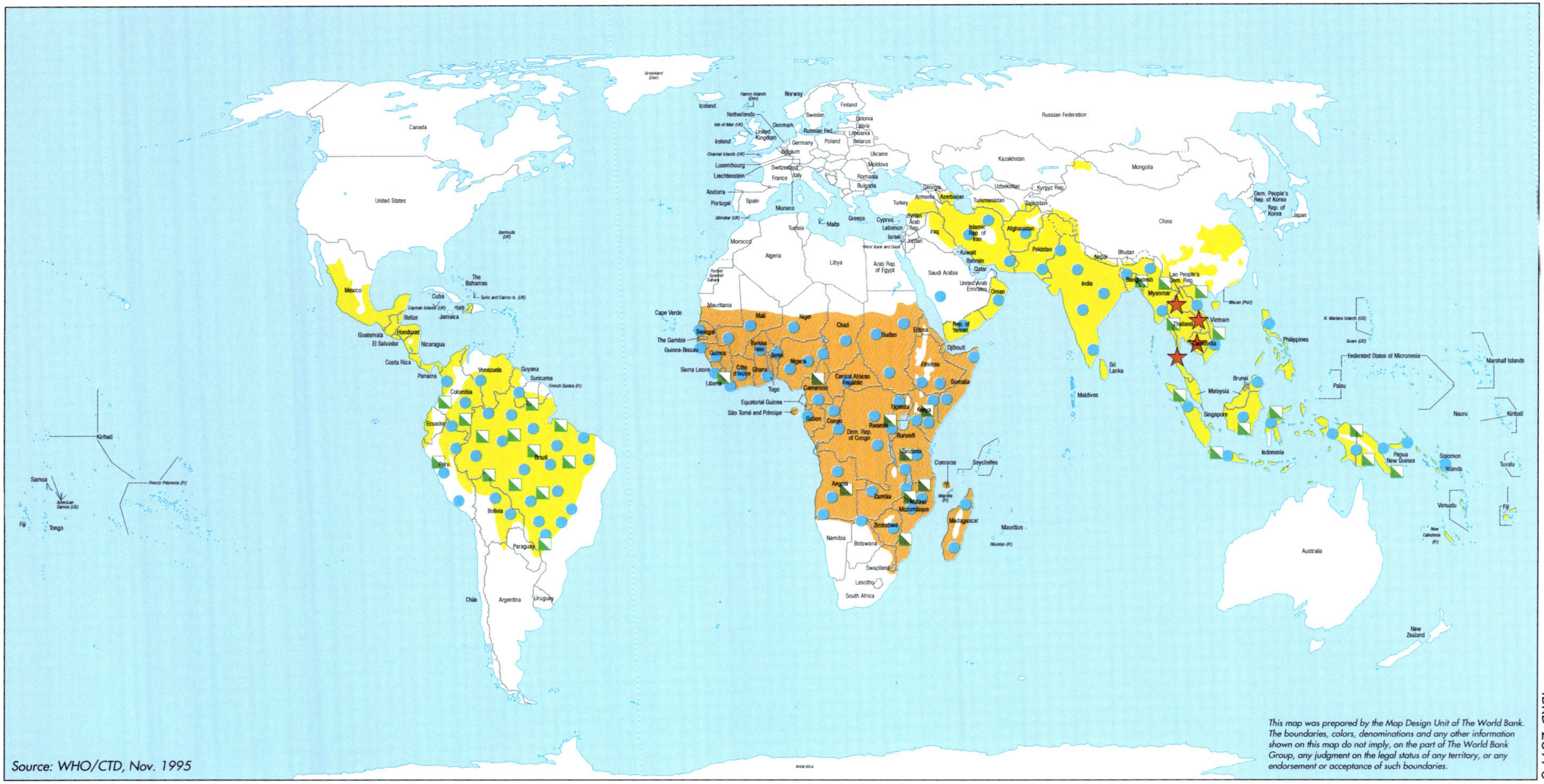

Source: WHO/CTD, Nov. 1995

This map was prepared by the Map Design Unit of The World Bank. The boundaries, colors, denominations and any other information shown on this map do not imply, on the part of The World Bank Group, any judgment on the legal status of any territory, or any endorsement or acceptance of such boundaries.

Health Expenditures as Percent of GDP

- Health expenditures 3% or less of GDP and health expenditures per capita less than $20
- 3% or less of GDP
- Between 3% and 6% of GDP
- 6% or more of GDP
- No data

IBRD 28975

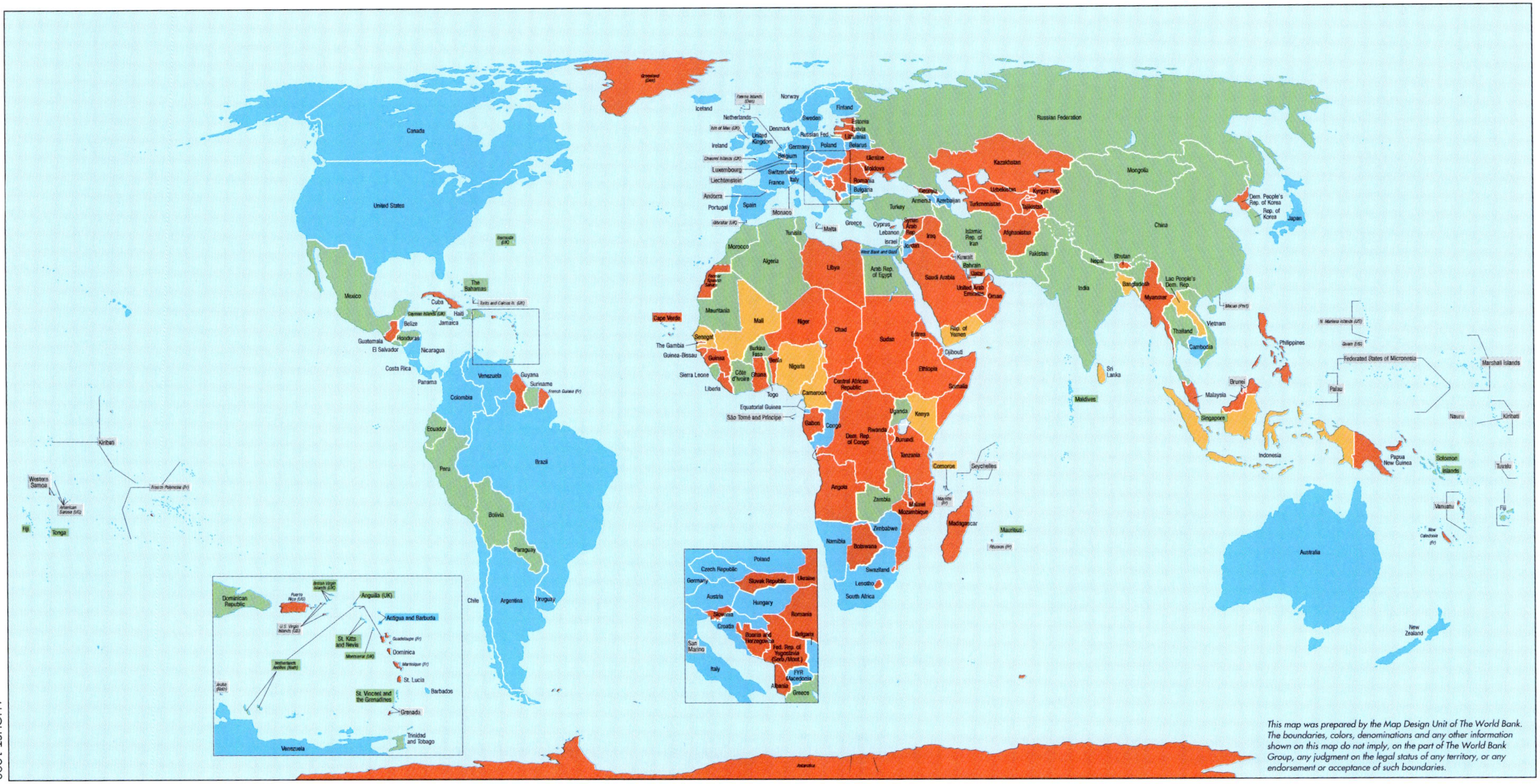

This map was prepared by the Map Design Unit of The World Bank. The boundaries, colors, denominations and any other information shown on this map do not imply, on the part of The World Bank Group, any judgment on the legal status of any territory, or any endorsement or acceptance of such boundaries.

AUGUST 1998

Active and Future World Bank/IDA Financed HNP Projects

Current IBRD Financed HNP Projects
Current IDA Financed HNP Projects
Pipeline HNP Projects: 1997 - 2000

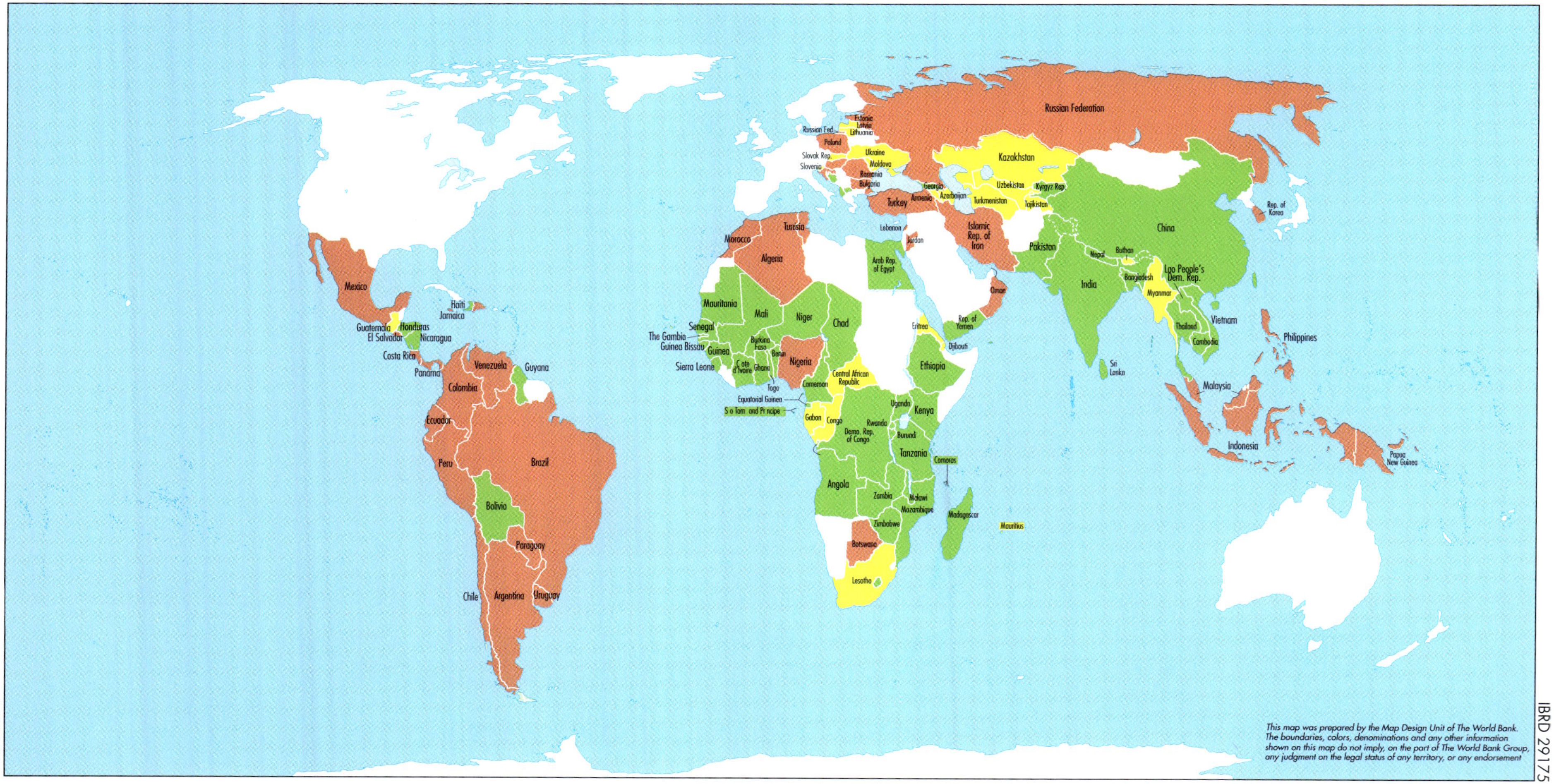

The World by Region

Low- and middle-income economies
- East Asia and the Pacific
- Europe and Central Asia
- Latin America and the Caribbean
- Middle East and North Africa
- South Asia
- Sub-Saharan Africa

High-income economies
- OECD
- Other

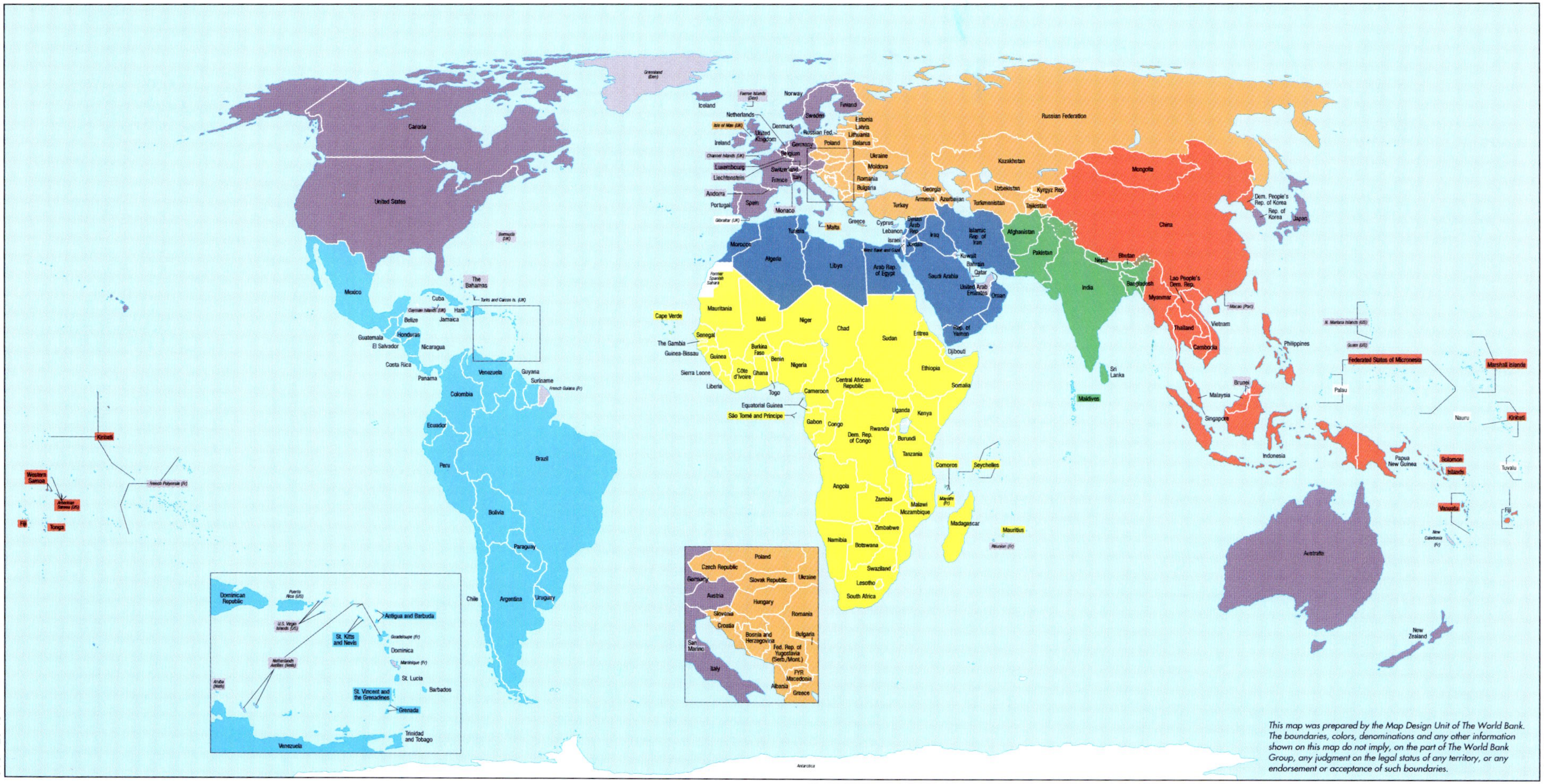

IBRD 28977

AUGUST 1998

Distributors of World Bank Publications

Prices and credit terms vary from country to country. Consult your local distributor before placing an order.

ARGENTINA
Oficina del Libro Internacional
Av. Cordoba 1877
1120 Buenos Aires
Tel: (54 1) 815-8354
Fax: (54 1) 815-8156

AUSTRALIA, FIJI, PAPUA NEW GUINEA, SOLOMON ISLANDS, VANUATU, AND WESTERN SAMOA
D.A. Information Services
648 Whitehorse Road
Mitcham 3132
Victoria
Tel: (61) 3 9210 7777
Fax: (61) 3 9210 7788
E-mail: service@dadirect.com.au
URL: http://www .dadirect.com.au

AUSTRIA
Gerold and Co.
Weihburggasse 26
A-1011 Wien
Tel: (43 1) 512-47-31-0
Fax: (43 1) 512-47-31-29
URL: http://www .gerold.co/at.online

BANGLADESH
Micro Industries Development Assistance Society (MIDAS)
House 5, Road 16
Dhanmondi R/Area
Dhaka 1209
Tel: (880 2) 326427
Fax: (880 2) 811188

BELGIUM
Jean De Lannoy
Av. du Roi 202
1060 Brussels
Tel: (32 2) 538-5169
Fax: (32 2) 538-0841

BRAZIL
Publicacões Tecnicas Internacionais Ltda.
Rua Peixoto Gomide, 209
01409 Sao Paulo, SP.
Tel: (55 11) 259-6644
Fax: (55 11) 258-6990
E-mail: postmaster@pti.uol.br
URL: http://www .uol.br

CANADA
Renouf Publishing Co. Ltd.
5369 Canotek Road
Ottawa, Ontario K1J 9J3
Tel: (613) 745-2665
Fax: (613) 745-7660
E-mail: order .dept@renoufbooks.com
URL: http:// www .renoufbooks.com

CHINA
China Financial & Economic Publishing House
8, Da Fo Si Dong Jie
Beijing
Tel: (86 10) 6333-8257
Fax: (86 10) 6401-7365

COLOMBIA
Infoenlace Ltda.
Carrera 6 No. 51-21
Apartado Aereo 34270
Santafé de Bogotá, D.C.
Tel: (57 1) 285-2798
Fax: (57 1) 285-2798

COTE D'IVOIRE
Center d'Edition et de Diffusion Africaines (CEDA)
04 B.P. 541
Abidjan 04
Tel: (225) 24 6510;24 6511
Fax: (225) 25 0567

CYPRUS
Center for Applied Research
Cyprus College
6, Diogenes Street, Engomi
P.O. Box 2006
Nicosia
Tel: (357 2) 44-1730
Fax: (357 2) 46-2051

CZECH REPUBLIC
National Information Center
prodejna, Konviktska 5
CS – 113 57 Prague 1
Tel: (42 2) 2422-9433
Fax: (42 2) 2422-1484
URL: http://www .nis.cz/

DENMARK
SamfundsLitteratur
Rosenoerns Allé 11
DK-1970 Frederiksberg C
Tel: (45 31) 351942
Fax: (45 31) 357822
URL: http://www.sl.cbs.dk

ECUADOR
Libri Mundi
Libreria Internacional
P.O. Box 17-01-3029
Juan Leon Mera 851
Quito
Tel: (593 2) 521-606
Fax: (593 2) 504-209
E-mail: librimu1@librimundi.com.ec
E-mail: librimu2@librimundi.com.ec

EGYPT, ARAB REPUBLIC OF
Al Ahram Distribution Agency
Al Galaa Street
Cairo
Tel: (20 2) 578-6083
Fax: (20 2) 578-6833

The Middle East Observer
41, Sherif Street
Cairo
Tel: (20 2) 393-9732
Fax: (20 2) 393-9732

FINLAND
Akateeminen Kirjakauppa
P.O. Box 128
FIN-00101 Helsinki
Tel: (358 0) 121-4418
Fax: (358 0) 121-4435
E-mail: akatilaus@stockmann.fi
URL: http://www .akateeminen.com/

FRANCE
World Bank Publications
66, avenue d'Iéna
75116 Paris
Tel: (33 1) 40-69-30-56/57
Fax: (33 1) 40-69-30-68

GERMANY
UNO-Verlag
Poppelsdorfer Allee 55
53115 Bonn
Tel: (49 228) 949020
Fax: (49 228) 217492
URL: http://www.uno-verlag.de
E-mail: unoverlag@aol.com

GREECE
Papasotiriou S.A.
35, Stournara Str.
106 82 Athens
Tel: (30 1) 364-1826
Fax: (30 1) 364-8254

HAITI
Culture Diffusion
5, Rue Capois
C.P. 257
Port-au-Prince
Tel: (509) 23 9260
Fax: (509) 23 4858

HONG KONG, MACAO
Asia 2000 Ltd.
Sales & Circulation Department
Seabird House, unit 1101-02
22-28 Wyndham Street, Central
Hong Kong
Tel: (852) 2530-1409
Fax: (852) 2526-1107
E-mail: sales@asia2000.com.hk
URL: http://www .asia2000.com.hk

HUNGARY
Euro Info Service
Margitszgeti Europa Haz
H-1138 Budapest
Tel: (36 1) 111 6061
Fax: (36 1) 302 5035
E-mail: euroinfo@mail.matav.hu

INDIA
Allied Publishers Ltd.
751 Mount Road
Madras - 600 002
Tel: (91 44) 852-3938
Fax: (91 44) 852-0649

INDONESIA
Pt. Indira Limited
Jalan Borobudur 20
P.O. Box 181
Jakarta 10320
Tel: (62 21) 390-4290
Fax: (62 21) 390-4289

IRAN
Ketab Sara Co. Publishers
Khaled Eslamboli Ave., 6th Street
Delafrooz Alley No. 8
P.O. Box 15745-733
Tehran 15117
Tel: (98 21) 8717819; 8716104
Fax: (98 21) 8712479
E-mail: ketab-sara@neda.net.ir

Kowkab Publishers
P.O. Box 19575-511
Tehran 15117
Tel: (98 21) 258-3723
Fax: (98 21) 258-3723

IRELAND
Government Supplies Agency
Oifig an tSoláthair
4-5 Harcourt Road
Dublin 2
Tel: (353 1) 661-3111
Fax: (353 1) 475-2670

ISRAEL
Yozmot Literature Ltd.
P.O. Box 56055
3 Yohanan Hasandlar Street
Tel Aviv 61560
Tel: (972 3) 5285-397
Fax: (972 3) 5285-397

R.O.Y. International
PO Box 13056
Tel Aviv 61130
Tel: (972 3) 5461423
Fax: (972 3) 5461442
E-mail: royil@netvision.net.il

Palestinian Authority/Middle East
Index Information Services
P.O.B. 19502 Jerusalem
Tel: (972 2) 6271219
Fax: (972 2) 6271634

ITALY
Licosa Commissionaria Sansoni SPA
Via Duca Di Calabria, 1/1
Casella Postale 552
50125 Firenze
Tel: (55) 645-415
Fax: (55) 641-257
E-mail: licosa@ftbcc.it
URL: http://www .ftbcc.it/licosa

JAMAICA
Ian Randle Publishers Ltd.
206 Old Hope Road
Kingston 6
Tel: 876-927-2085
Fax: 876-977-0243
E-mail: irpl@colis.com

JAPAN
Eastern Book Service
3-13 Hongo 3-chome, Bunkyo-ku
Tokyo 113
Tel: (81 3) 3818-0861
Fax: (81 3) 3818-0864
E-mail: orders@svt-ebs.co.jp
URL: http://www.bekkoame.or.jp/~svt-ebs

KENYA
Africa Book Service (E.A.) Ltd.
Quaran House, Mfangano Street
P.O. Box 45245
Nairobi
Tel: (254 2) 223 641
Fax: (254 2) 330 272

KOREA, REPUBLIC OF
Daejon Trading Co. Ltd.
P.O. Box 34, Youida
706 Seoun Bldg.
44-6 Youido-Dong, Yeongchengpo-Ku
Seoul
Tel: (82 2) 785-1631/4
Fax: (82 2) 784-0315

MALAYSIA
University of Malaya Cooperative
Bookshop, Limited
P.O. Box 1127
Jalan Pantai Baru
59700 Kuala Lumpur
Tel: (60 3) 756-5000
Fax: (60 3) 755-4424

MEXICO
INFOTEC
Av. San Fernando No. 37
Col. Toriello Guerra
14050 Mexico, D.F.
Tel: (52 5) 624-2800
Fax: (52 5) 624-2822
E-mail: infotec@rtn.net.mx
URL: http://rtn.net.mx

NEPAL
Everest Media International
Services (P.) Ltd.
GPO Box 5443
Kathmandu
Tel: (977 1) 472 152
Fax: (977 1) 224 431

NETHERLANDS
De Lindeboom/InOr-Publikaties
P.O. Box 202
7480 AE Haaksbergen
Tel: (31 53) 574-0004
Fax: (31 53) 572-9296
E-mail: lindeboo@worldonline.nl
URL: http://www .worldonline.nl/~lindeboo

NEW ZEALAND
EBSCO NZ Ltd.
Private Mail Bag 99914, New Market
Auckland
Tel: (64 9) 524-8119
Fax: (64 9) 524-8067

NIGERIA
University Press Limited
Three Crowns Building Jericho
Private Mail Bag 5095
Ibadan
Tel: (234 22) 41-1356
Fax: (234 22) 41-2056

NORWAY
NIC Info A/S
Book Department
Postboks 6512 Etterstad
N-0606 Oslo
Tel: (47 22) 97-4500
Fax: (47 22) 97-4545

PAKISTAN
Mirza Book Agency
65, Shahrah-e-Quaid-e-Azam
Lahore 54000
Tel: (92 42) 735 3601
Fax: (92 42) 576 3714

Oxford University Press
5 Bangalore Town
Sharae Faisal
PO Box 13033
Karachi-75350
Tel: (92 21) 446307
Fax: (92 21) 4547640
E-mail: ouppak@TheOffice.net

Pak Book Corporation
Aziz Chambers 21
Queen's Road
Lahore
Tel: (92 42) 636 3222; 636 0885
Fax: (92 42) 636 2328
E-mail: pbc@brain.net.pk

PERU
Editorial Desarrollo SA
Apartado 3824
Lima 1
Tel: (51 14) 285380
Fax: (51 14) 286628

PHILIPPINES
International Booksource Center Inc.
1127-A Antipolo St.
Barangay, Venezuela
Makati City
Tel: (63 2) 896 6501; 6505; 6507
Fax: (63 2) 896 1741

POLAND
International Publishing Service
Ul. Piekna 31/37
00-677 Warzawa
Tel: (48 2) 628-6089
Fax: (48 2) 621-7255
E-mail: books%ips@ikp.atm.com.pl
URL: http://www .ipscg.waw.pl/ips/export/

PORTUGAL
Livraria Portugal
Apartado 2681
Rua Do Carmo 70-74
1200 Lisbon
Tel: (1) 347-4982
Fax: (1) 347-0264

ROMANIA
Compani De Librarii Bucuresti S.A.
Str. Lipscani no. 26, sector 3
Bucharest
Tel: (40 1) 613 9645
Fax: (40 1) 312 4000

RUSSIAN FEDERATION
Isdatelstvo <Ves Mir>
9a, Lolpachniy Pereulok
Moscow 101831
Tel: (7 095) 917 87 49
Fax: (7 095) 917 92 59

SINGAPORE, TAIWAN, MYANMAR, BRUNEI
Asahgate Publishing Asia
Pacific Pte. Ltd.
41 Kallang Pudding Road #04-03
Golden Wheel Building
Singapore 349316
Tel: (65) 741-5166
Fax: (65) 742-9356
E-mail: ashgate@asianconnect.com

SLOVENIA
Gospodarski Vestnik Publishing Grp.
Dunajska cesta 5
1000 Ljubljana
Tel: (386 61) 133 83 47; 132 12 30
Fax: (386 61) 133 80 30
E-mail: repansekj@gvestnik.si

SOUTH AFRICA, BOTSWANA
For single titles:
Oxford University Press
Southern Africa
Vasco Boulevard, Goodwood
P.O. Box 12119
N1 City 7463
Cape Town
Tel: (27 21) 595-440
Fax: (27 21) 595-4430
E-mail: oxford@oup.co.za

For subscription orders:
International Subscription Service
P.O. Box 41095, Craighall
Johannesburg 2024
Tel: (27 11) 880-1448
Fax: (27 11) 880-6248
E-mail: iss@is.co.za

SPAIN
Mundi-Prensa Libros, S.A.
Castello 37
28001 Madrid
Tel: (34 1) 431-3399
Fax: (34 1) 575-3998
E-mail: libreria@mundiprensa.es
URL: http://www .mundiprensa.es/

Mundi-Prensa Barcelona
Consell de Cent, 391
08009 Barcelona
Tel: (34 3) 488-3492
Fax: (34 3) 487-7659
E-mail: barcelona@mundiprensa.es

SRI LANKA, THE MALDIVES
Lake House Bookshop
100, Sir Chittampalam Gardiner
Mawatha
Colombo 2
Tel: (94 1) 32105
Fax: (94 1) 432104
E-mail: LHL@sri.lanka.net

SWEDEN
Wennergren-Williams AB
P. O. Box 1305
S-171 25 Solna
Tel: (46 8) 705-97-50
Fax: (46 8) 27-00-71
E-mail: mail@wwi.se

SWITZERLAND
Librairie Payot
Service Institutionnel
Côtes-de-Montbenon 30
1002 Lausanne
Tel: (41 21) 341-3229
Fax: (41 21) 341-3235

ADECO Van Diermen Editions
Techniques
Ch. de Lacuez 41
CH1807 Blonay
Tel: (41 21) 943 2673
Fax: (41 21) 943 3605

THAILAND
Central Books Distribution
306 Silom Road
Bangkok 10500
Tel: (66 2) 235-5400
Fax: (66 2) 237-8321

TRINIDAD & TOBAGO, AND THE CARRIBBEAN
Systematics Studies Unit
9 Watts Street, Curepe
Trinidad, West Indies
Tel: (809) 662-5654
Fax: (809) 662-5654
E-mail: tobe@trinidad.net

UGANDA
Gustro Ltd.
PO Box 9997, Madhvani Building
Plot 16/4 Jinja Rd.
Kampala
Tel: (256 41) 251 467
Fax: (256 41) 251 468
E-mail: gus@swiftuganda.com

UNITED KINGDOM
Microinfo Ltd.
P.O. Box 3
Alton, Hampshire GU34 2PG
England
Tel: (44 1420) 86848
Fax: (44 1420) 89889
E-mail:wbank@ukminfo.demon.co.uk
URL: http://www .microinfo.co.uk

VENEZUELA
Tecni-Ciencia Libros, S.A.
Centro Cuidad Comercial Tamanco
Nivel C2
Caracas
Tel: (58 2) 959 5547; 5035; 0016
Fax: (58 2) 959 5636

ZAMBIA
University Bookshop
University of Zambia
Great East Road Campus
P.O. Box 32379
Lusaka
Tel: (260 1) 252 576
Fax: (260 1) 253 952

ZIMBABWE
Longman Zimbabwe (Pvt.)Ltd.
Tourle Road, Ardbennie
P.O. Box ST125
Southerton
Harare
Tel: (263 4) 6216617
Fax: (263 4) 621670